Understanding Alzheimer's Disease

Understanding Alzheimer's Disease

**Neal R. Cutler, M.D., and
John J. Sramek, Pharm.D.**

California Clinical Trials, Beverly Hills, California
International Clinical Trials, London, England

Understanding Health and Sickness Series, Miriam Bloom, Editor
University Press of Mississippi
Jackson

Copyright © 1996 by the University Press of Mississippi
All rights reserved
Manufactured in the United States of America
99 98 97 96   4 3 2 1
The paper in this book meets the guidelines for permanence and dura-
bility of the Committee on Production Guidelines for Book Longevity of
the Council on Library Resources.

Illustrations by Regan Causey Tuder

Library of Congress Cataloging-in-Publication Data

Cutler, Neal R.
    Understanding Alzheimer's disease / Neal R. Cutler and John J.
  Sramek.
        p.   cm.—(Understanding health and sickness series)
    Includes index.
    ISBN 0-87805-910-5 (cloth : alk. paper).—ISBN 0-87805-911-3 (pbk. :
  alk. paper)
    1. Alzheimer's disease.   I. Sramek, John J.   II. Title.   III. Series.
  RC523.C885   1996
  616.8'31—dc20   96-20284
                                                             CIP

British Library Cataloging-in-Publication data available

Contents

Dedication and Acknowledgments

We dedicate this book to all Alzheimer's patients and their families and caregivers. Thanks to their overwhelming willingness to participate in research, future generations may not have to suffer from this devastating illness.

We are indebted to Giedra Miller for assistance in outlining, researching, and writing the manuscript. Paul A. Smith reviewed early drafts of chapters 3 and 6 and offered valuable suggestions, and Dr. Neil M. Kurtz provided useful feedback on a later manuscript. We also thank our editor, Dr. Miriam Bloom. Her many helpful comments and boundless patience made writing this book a true pleasure.

Introduction

> The Immortals of Luggnagg "have no remem-
> brance of anything but what they learned and ob-
> served in their youth [and] forget the common ap-
> pellation of things, and the names of persons, even
> of . . . nearest friends and relations. . . . For the same
> reason they never can amuse themselves with reading,
> because their memory will not serve to carry them
> from the beginning of a sentence to the end. . . . Nei-
> ther are they able . . . to hold any conversation (far-
> ther than a few general words) with their neighbors."
>
> —Gulliver's account of a race of
> immortal people in Jonathan Swift's
> *Gulliver's Travels*

It is likely that the Immortals of Luggnagg would be diagnosed today as having Alzheimer's disease. In creating and
describing the characteristics of this race, Swift may not have
had to look far. Dementia was well known in his day, and in
fact has been described from ancient times. The Greek judge
Solon (500 B.C.E.) sought to protect the rights of the mentally
impaired by requiring that wills not be made by anyone under the influence of "physical pain, violence, old age, or the
persuasion of a woman." Approximately 100 years later in *The
Republic*, Plato recognized the loss of capacity in some aged
people when he wrote that certain crimes could be excused
if committed in a state of madness, disease, or extreme old
age. In the first century B.C.E., the poet Lucretius sang of
dementia: "[W]hen the mighty force of years their frame hath
shaken and their limbs collapse with blunted strength, the
intellect grows dim. The tongue talks nonsense, and the mind
gives way. All things fail, and all together go." Shakespeare's
King Lear suffered some sort of dementing illness, too.

Most of these old accounts seem to consider dementia and
memory loss an expected part of aging rather than a disease

process. Only in the last 100 years have we begun to change this view, thanks to the rapid pace of research on Alzheimer's disease and other types of dementias that has provided wholly new ways of looking at memory loss and aging. Though many people continue to believe that severe memory loss is inevitable, this is simply not so. Minor memory loss, on the other hand, such as the occasional forgetting of car keys or the names of seldom-seen acquaintances, is a normal part of aging for everyone and is not cause for concern. People expect their bodies and reflexes to slow down with age, but not their brains. Physicians now recognize that even healthy people are less able to remember certain types of information as they get older. These minor memory lapses, which often involve matters of little importance that are usually remembered later on, are evidence of "age-associated memory impairment." This type of memory loss is most apparent when someone is under pressure.

Memory loss can also be caused by various life stressors including fatigue, grief, depression, illness, certain medications, and vision or hearing loss, or by a lack of concentration. Such losses can occur at any age and can be reversed when the stress lets up. People can improve their memory preservation by cutting back on alcohol, eating well-balanced meals, and making sure medications are used only when necessary and taken as directed.

Distinguishing normal memory loss from dementia is mostly a matter of evaluating the impact of the memory loss on normal functioning. Most people with normal memory loss can compensate by writing reminders to themselves, making lists, allowing more time for remembering, or repeating out loud the information they want to remember, and their impairment rarely worsens over time. In contrast, memory loss associated with dementia is progressive and disabling, interfering more and more with normal daily activities as time goes by. "Forgetfulness" that seems to be causing a lot of serious problems is abnormal and likely the result of a disease.

At one time, all people over the age of 65 who exhibited this type of severe memory loss were said to suffer from *senile dementia,* and those afflicted with similar symptoms at younger ages were said to have *pre-senile dementia.* Today these labels have largely been dropped, and *dementia* is most commonly used to describe any loss of intellectual function, including thinking, remembering, and reasoning, that is severe enough to interfere with normal activities. Dementia is not a disease in itself but a group of symptoms that may accompany certain diseases or conditions. Alzheimer's disease is one of the most common causes of dementia, but there are others, several of which are reversible. Anyone who starts to show any signs of dementia should get a comprehensive medical evaluation to determine its cause.

The first signs of Alzheimer's disease include difficulty in remembering recent events and performing familiar everyday tasks. As the disease progresses, the affected person may experience confusion, personality and behavior changes, impaired judgment, and difficulty finding words, finishing thoughts, or following directions. These changes occur at widely varying speeds in different people, and not all changes occur in everyone, but the outcome is always the same. Eventually, people with Alzheimer's disease completely lose the ability to care for themselves and must be confined to bed with constant care. In the latest stages of disease the brain can no longer regulate body functions, and victims die of malnutrition, dehydration, infection, heart failure, or other complications. Unfortunately, science has not yet found a cure.

Though Alzheimer's disease has probably been around as long as we have been *Homo sapiens,* it is only now reaching epidemic proportions as our society enjoys increased longevity. The first description of what we now know as Alzheimer's disease appeared in the medical literature in 1907. The case of pre-senile dementia that Dr. Alois Alzheimer described involved a 51-year-old woman whose memory and personality deteriorated gradually while she simultaneously

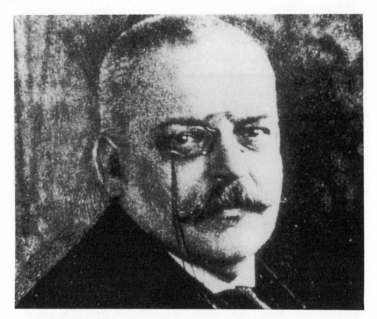

FIG I.1. Dr. Alois Alzheimer (1864–1915)

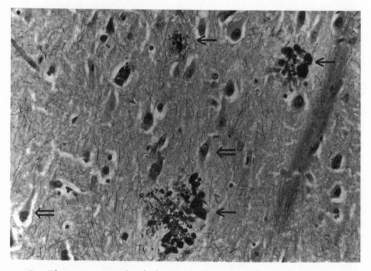

FIG I.2. Photomicrograph of plaques and tangles. The three plaques in the figure are marked by single arrows (←), and two of the numerous tangles are marked by double arrows(⇐).

developed problems understanding, speaking, and writing (fig. I.1). After the woman's death, Alzheimer found tangles of neuron (nerve) fibers and deposits of a peculiar substance—the Alzheimer plaque—in her brain (fig. I.2). Though the neuronal tangles had been seen before in older demented people, their appearance in such a young person, along with the unusual deposits, prompted Alzheimer to suggest that the disease represented a new form of dementia. His colleague Emil Kraepelin agreed, and named it *Morbus Alzheimer*, or Alzheimer's disease. Having shown that neurofibrillary tangles and Alzheimer plaques, the primary distinguishing features of Alzheimer's disease, may appear in patients of any age, modern neuropathologists dropped the distinction between presenile and senile dementia that had been favored by Alzheimer. While early onset of Alzheimer's is quite unsettling and even more devastating to patient and family than a case that begins later in life, the disease in both cases is essentially the same.

Alzheimer's disease has received growing attention in the years since it was first described, in large part because the affected population is growing. Americans 65 or older numbered 3 million in 1900; now there are over 27 million, and government figures predict that over 50 million Americans will be 65 or older in the year 2030. People over 75 are the fastest-growing segment of the population in the United States. And because people over the age of 75 require more health and social services, this increased longevity translates to greater social and economic costs, particularly because the prevalence of Alzheimer's disease rises so steeply with age. While it is difficult to determine precisely how common Alzheimer's disease is, typical estimates are about 0.5 percent of people aged 65 years, rising to 3 percent of 75-year-olds and 10 percent of 85-year-olds. The risk of a person's developing the disease seems to be about 1 to 2 chances in 100 by the age of 65, rising to a 1 in 5 chance by age 80. It is important to keep these figures in perspective, however; 4 out of 5 people over 80 have normal or nearly normal cognitive functioning.

The only clearly delineated risk factor for Alzheimer's disease is age; prevalence rises exponentially with advancing years. Researchers have also found evidence that people who carry a gene for a particular protein, *apolipoprotein E4* (see chapter 3), are at significantly greater risk for developing Alzheimer's disease than people who carry genes for other forms of the protein. Not all people with the gene develop Alzheimer's disease, however, and not all people with the disease carry the gene. There are more forces at work than just the action of one gene. Other suggested risk factors are more controversial. For example, some studies have shown that Alzheimer's disease is more common in women than in men. There is some speculation that this conclusion is the result of the presence of fewer men in the sample tested or of women's living longer and thus appearing affected more often, since incidence rises with age. There is also some evidence to suggest that education has a protective effect; people with higher education are less likely to develop Alzheimer's disease than people who had only a primary education. It appears likely that education does not actually prevent Alzheimer's disease but delays its onset by up to 5 years, though further research is necessary to confirm this hypothesis. Similarly, jobs or other life activities that provide mental challenges seem to have a protective effect.

This book was written for anyone interested in learning more about Alzheimer's disease—people with the disease and their families and caregivers; professionals who might serve Alzheimer's patients, including nurses, lawyers, accountants, and social workers; teachers; and anyone else curious to know exactly what goes on in Alzheimer's, a disease that seems to get mentioned every time someone forgets something. We begin with a description of the course of Alzheimer's disease, from early to advanced stages, giving a broad picture of what behaviors and medical problems can be expected when someone has the disease. This chapter includes a detailed discussion of current procedures used to diagnose Alzheimer's disease. While diagnosis is never definite until plaques and tangles have been found in brain tissue during an autopsy, diagnostic accuracy in life has increased greatly in recent years. This is because physicians have become more familiar with Alzheimer's disease and its characteristic signs, and because technology that can recognize certain other common causes of dementia, such as strokes, has improved.

In chapter 2 we offer a brief discussion of normal functioning of the brain in an effort to permit greater understanding of the disease processes that are seen in Alzheimer's and how they lead to symptoms. Chapter 3 focuses on various theories about the causes of Alzheimer's disease. We review older theories that are no longer in favor and then discuss evidence that Alzheimer's is a genetic disease. The changes that occur in the brain are then described in full, and various possibilities for the origin of plaques and tangles and other related problems are presented.

In the fourth chapter we discuss what is involved in caring for people with Alzheimer's disease. Because so many people continue to live at home under the care of family members until the final stages of the disease, we begin by discussing how to care for patients at home, including important communication techniques for all those who come in contact with Alzheimer's patients. We follow this up with recommendations for finding outside services to help care for people with Alzheimer's disease, including adult day care and long-term residential care programs, and we offer suggestions for handling legal and financial matters.

The fifth chapter reviews all the treatments currently available for Alzheimer's disease. Most of the existing treatments alleviate some of the troublesome behaviors seen in the disease but do little to correct memory and thought problems. One important exception to this is tacrine (Cognex), a drug that was recently approved for use in Alzheimer's disease. It appears to improve cognitive functioning in perhaps a third of patients who try it for at least several months.

The last twenty years have seen a great surge in research devoted to finding treatments and/or cures for Alzheimer's disease. The final chapter describes this research, beginning with a general description of how drugs and treatments are developed (this may be useful to people with Alzheimer's disease who are asked to participate in research studies). We explain why it takes so long to find drugs that work and then describe several of the main lines of research that provide hope for the future. Although the exact cause of Alzheimer's disease is still unknown, the flood of research during the last 20 years has revealed so much about the progression of the disease that beneficial treatments are likely to begin appearing in the near future and to continue improving with time.

Understanding Alzheimer's Disease

1. What Happens When Someone Gets Alzheimer's Disease? Course of Disease and Diagnosis

It is often difficult to determine exactly when someone gets Alzheimer's disease, because the disease sets in so gradually that changes are nearly imperceptible. Typically several years pass before a person is brought in for evaluation. The rate of progression from milder to more severe stages is gradual and differs from individual to individual. People who have a relatively early disease onset (say, in their fifties) often deteriorate more rapidly than those whose onset is later in life.

During the early stages of the disease, people suffer from memory impairment so mild that few people will notice. Loss of word-finding ability is commonly the first language difficulty reported in the disease, and at first this is only noticeable for infrequently used words or words with multiple or subtle meanings. Despite this difficulty and the occasional omission of meaningful words, people in the early stages of Alzheimer's disease are generally able to communicate effectively using correct grammar and syntax. Patients may forget seldom-used names of distant acquaintances, phone numbers, and conversations or details of recent events, and may misplace keys or other items, but often these lapses go unnoticed by observers.

As the disease progresses, people with Alzheimer's disease have a hard time finding the right words, and they speak with growing reluctance. It becomes more difficult for them to pay attention, to reason, and to understand abstract concepts. For example, they may experience minor difficulties with calculations, such as those required to balance a checkbook or estimate how much a cartload of groceries costs, and they may have difficulty understanding complex or new ideas. They begin to lose their ability to operate appliances and must be assisted, and they may also begin to drive less safely. At some point patients become disoriented in time and place so they often need to be reminded what day it is or be given directions to get to places that were once familiar. Furthermore, the personalities of people in the early stages of Alzheimer's disease may change subtly. They may show indifference, lack of initiative, or passivity. A once-talkative person may become quiet or withdrawn, or a mild-mannered, compassionate person may appear to be indifferent, insensitive, or aggressive.

On the whole, however, someone in the mild stages of Alzheimer's disease will generally retain normal social skills, basic self-care abilities, and neurological function. To a casual observer, this person will appear normal. Patients, too, may experience impaired insight such that they are unaware of their deficits. It is usually family members or close friends who most clearly notice the changes and insist upon medical evaluation. People with Alzheimer's disease may be fairly well along in the disease before such an evaluation takes place. If they do realize the extent of their deficits, they may experience a great deal of sadness in what is essentially a grieving process. Such feelings are normal and to be expected. A smaller proportion of people with Alzheimer's may suffer bouts of more serious forms of depression, usually in the early-to-middle stages of the disease.

In the middle stages of Alzheimer's disease, comprehension of written and spoken language deteriorates further, especially when complex topics are involved, though comprehension is by and large better than expression. People with moderate Alzheimer's disease still generally use correct grammar, and speech often remains fluent, but sentence fragments and meaningless statements become more common, as do empty, made-up, or sound-alike words. They may begin to repeat ideas in conversation or incessantly repeat phrases or questions. Furthermore, affected individuals are easily distracted and may often digress, spending much time on reliable topics from the past. They may begin to show lack of sensitivity regarding conversational situations and participants, raising touchy subjects in front of children or in situations where such subjects are not appropriate, or repeatedly swearing or making tactless remarks without awareness of their impact. Nevertheless, people with moderate Alzheimer's disease generally know when they are expected to talk and can recognize questions. They are likely to withdraw in difficult social situations, such as when there are many people involved in a discussion. They may fail to greet newcomers, and they are less likely to correct themselves when they use a wrong word.

As vocabulary is reduced further along in the disease, Alzheimer's patients will begin to use more empty words like "thing" and "stuff," and may begin to rely on roundabout ways of expressing themselves (for example, substituting "that stuff I use for washing" for "soap" or "the metal thing on my finger" for "ring"), though in early stages they may correct themselves when they are able. Most people can still correctly use social phrases like "goodbye," "how are you," and "nice to meet you," but they gradually lose their ability to produce series of related, meaningful sentences. They begin to show difficulties comprehending new information and any kind of abstract information, including humor, sarcasm, and nonliteral statements. They may show signs of frustration with their inability to communicate, becoming angry or argumentative. Other personality changes may surface, such as a tendency to become hypochondriacal (preoccupied with health) or to show discomfort in social activities.

In the moderate-to-severe stages of Alzheimer's disease, memory of recent events becomes seriously compromised. Patients begin to show disorientation and cannot distinguish between day and night. They can no longer handle money or make simple purchases. Their functions at home become progressively restricted as it becomes more and more difficult for them to perform simple chores such as setting the table or washing dishes. They begin to lose physical coordination, needing assistance in dressing and grooming and occasionally having balance problems. Troublesome behaviors frequently complicate the management of disease at this point and lead to patients being put in nursing homes. Such behaviors include suspiciousness, delusions (thinking a misplaced item has been stolen or believing a spouse has been unfaithful, for example), misperceptions, hyperactivity, restlessness and wandering, verbal and physical aggression, and hallucinations. Sometimes these behaviors stem from patients' acting out memories from their early life. For example, someone who lived on a farm in childhood might rise in the middle of the night to check the chicken coop outside; while the caregiver interprets this as problematic wandering and installs new locks on the doors, the patient may believe the action is an important task that must be accomplished.

Another major problem at this stage is incontinence. People with Alzheimer's disease can no longer connect the bodily sensation of needing to go to the bathroom with the knowledge of what they should do, or they may know but have trouble locating the bathroom. In any case, incontinence is one of the most common reasons for putting someone in a nursing home.

In the most advanced stages of the disease, Alzheimer's patients become totally dependent on their caregivers. Language deteriorates both in comprehension and output, and patients have even more difficulty comprehending new or complex information. Abstract ideas are completely incomprehensible at this point. Some people become mute, and most do not understand anything going on around them. Eventually the brain loses its ability to regulate body functions. Patients become bedridden and generally die of illnesses that are common in people confined to bed, such as exhaustion and/or weight loss from malnutrition, dehydration, pneumonia, urinary tract infections, or heart failure. The time between initial emergence of symptoms and death is highly variable from person to person but averages from 8 to 10 years. On average, Alzheimer's disease is diagnosed when a person is 78, two-and-a-half years after symptom onset at age 75.

As is apparent from this description, Alzheimer's disease is characterized overall by progressive memory loss and the decline of other mental functions such as attention, language, and reasoning ability. This decline is probably a result of the degeneration of nerve cells in the parts of the brain that are involved in thinking and remembering. Two characteristic features are found in these parts of the brain in people with Alzheimer's disease: neurofibrillary tangles, which are jumbled-up assemblages of the proteins that normally make up the outer layer of nerve cells in the brain, and neuritic plaques, which are complex deposits of several types of protein, most notably one called amyloid (see figures in the introduction and chapter 3). The only reliable way to diagnose Alzheimer's disease is to examine brain tissue under a microscope for the presence of these features, and this can only be done upon autopsy. Researchers trying to develop a lab test for the disease are making progress (see chapter 6), but so far there is no definitive test.

Thus doctors must rely upon other kinds of criteria to determine whether someone who comes for evaluation with signs of dementia has Alzheimer's disease. In particular, the diagnosis of Alzheimer's disease depends on ruling out other causes of dementia. With careful diagnosis and use of modern techniques and assessments, the diagnosis of Alzheimer's disease can be made in the doctor's office with nearly as much certainty as it can be made based on autopsy findings. Following are other causes of dementia and dementia-like symptoms, which must be ruled out:

Multi-infarct dementia (sometimes called *cerebrovascular* or just *vascular dementia*) is mental deterioration caused by multiple strokes in the brain. A stroke occurs when a blood clot gets lodged in an artery in the brain, blocking the flow of blood past the clot, or when the arteries in the brain harden (atherosclerosis) to the extent that blood cannot flow through. In either case, if the blockage does not let up, the nerve cells in the area of the brain not receiving blood will die. The area of tissue that dies is called an *infarct*; hence the name multi-infarct dementia.

The onset of this type of dementia may be sudden, because a number of small strokes can occur before there are any symptoms. Progression tends to be stepwise, with people sometimes improving between strokes. Because the strokes are small and localized, they damage only particular areas of the brain, and different areas may be affected each time. Eventually patients show disorientation, confusion, and behavioral changes in addition to intellectual deficits. Risk factors include high blood pressure, vascular disease, diabetes, and previous strokes. Recognition of the underlying condition (e.g., high blood pressure) can permit treatment, which may halt progression of the disease, though any brain damage already there cannot be cured or reversed.

People with *Parkinson's disease* do not produce enough *dopamine* in certain areas of the brain. Dopamine is a chemical in the brain that controls muscle activity in the nervous system. Characteristics of this disease are shaky movements (usually called tremors), stiffness, slowness, slow speech, and difficulty in the initiation of movement. These problems are often called parkinsonian symptoms even when they are seen in other illnesses, because they were originally associated with Parkinson's disease. More generally they are called *motor symptoms*—changes in the ability to control movements. Late in the course of Parkinson's, people may also show signs of dementia. Some Parkinson's patients develop Alzheimer's disease, and some Alzheimer's patients experience parkinsonian symptoms as part of their illness. Drugs can improve the motor symptoms of this disorder, but they do not improve the mental changes.

Huntington's disease is a hereditary disease that shows up in mid-life. It is characterized by involuntary movements of limbs and/or facial muscles and by a gradual intellectual decline. Personality changes are also common. The pattern of memory impairment is quite different from that in Alzheimer's disease. As the disease progresses, movements become severe and uncontrollable, and mental capacity may deteriorate to dementia. Huntington's disease is diagnosed by family history, recognition of the appropriate motor disorders, brain scans, and genetic testing. There are drugs that can treat the movement disorders and psychiatric symptoms in part, but nothing halts the progression of the disease, and it is ultimately fatal.

Creutzfeldt-Jakob disease is a rare fatal brain disease caused by a transmissible infectious agent, most likely a virus. It is characterized by failing memory, behavioral changes, and a lack of coordination early on in its progression. It works rapidly, usually causing death within one year of diagnosis. There is no known treatment.

Pick's disease, another rare brain disease, closely resembles Alzheimer's disease except at autopsy. Also, personality, behavior, and orientation changes tend to come before memory loss in Pick's disease, whereas the opposite is true for Alzheimer's disease.

In addition to the above-named irreversible disorders that can cause dementia, there are several disorders that can cause symptoms of dementia that are reversible or treatable. For example, *normal pressure hydrocephalus* is an uncommon disorder characterized by difficulty in walking, dementia, and urinary incontinence. It arises when an obstruction in the normal flow of spinal fluid causes a build-up of fluid in the brain. Factors contributing to the likelihood of contracting this disorder include a head injury or a history of meningitis or encephalitis. The condition may be treated by a neurosurgical procedure called a shunt, which diverts the built-up fluid away from the brain. This generally alleviates the symptoms of the disorder.

Depression is a psychiatric disorder characterized by sadness, inactivity, difficulty in thinking and concentration, feelings of hopelessness, and suicidal tendencies in some people.

Many severely depressed people experience mental deficits, and many demented people also suffer from depression. A number of effective treatments for depression can be useful in alleviating certain problems associated with dementia. Other problems that may cause symptoms of dementia include Lou Gehrig's disease (more formally known as *amyotrophic lateral sclerosis*), Wernicke-Korsakoff syndrome, multiple sclerosis, AIDS (in the latest stages), thyroid disorders, nutritional deficiencies, infections, syphilis, meningitis, alcoholism, brain tumors, head injuries, and adverse reactions to medications that can produce acute states of confusion (drug-induced organic brain syndromes).

A study examining the causes of dementia in people over 65 found that Alzheimer's disease was responsible 56 percent of the time, with other causes as follows: multi-infarct dementia, 14 percent; multiple causes, 12 percent; Parkinson's disease, 8 percent; brain injury, 4 percent; and other, 6 percent. Overlapping diseases become more common with advancing age, so that many people with symptoms of dementia have more than one dementing disorder. Most people with *mixed dementia* (dementia from multiple causes) have Alzheimer's disease in addition to some other disorder, such that Alzheimer's contributes to dementia in approximately 70 percent of demented patients over 65. Misdiagnosis or overdiagnosis of dementia is also common because of misinterpretation of mild brain scan findings and inaccurate diagnosis of depression as dementia.

Over the years, researchers have developed many sets of criteria for doctors to use when evaluating whether someone has Alzheimer's disease. One of the best was written by The Work Group on the Diagnosis of Alzheimer's Disease, established by the National Institute of Neurological and Communicative Disorders and Stroke (NINCDS) and the Alzheimer Disease and Related Disorders Association (ADRDA).[1] The NINCDS-ADRDA criteria, as they are known, were originally intended for use by researchers who wanted to ensure that people used in studies would all have the same kind of dementia. This is important because a treatment designed for Alzheimer's disease might not work in people who don't have it, and might appear less useful than it actually is if the study includes subjects who have other forms of dementia. The criteria have indeed proven useful for selecting subjects for research studies, but they are also used in traditional medical settings now because they provide a systematic approach to diagnosis that incorporates medical history and physical, neurological, neuropsychological, and psychiatric examinations.

The NINCDS-ADRDA document gives separate definitions for dementia and for Alzheimer's disease. *Dementia* is defined as progressive and global memory loss accompanied by deterioration of other intellectual functions including deficits in at least two of the following areas: language use, perception, motor skills, learning ability, problem-solving, abstract thought, and judgment. *Alzheimer's disease* is defined as the condition of having dementia with onset between ages 40 and 90, an absence of systemic or other brain diseases that could account for dementia, and a lack of disturbance in consciousness (see appendix A). Alzheimer's disease is further defined according to the certainty of diagnosis: "possible," "probable," or "definite." *Possible Alzheimer's disease* is diagnosed if the person's symptoms match the characteristics of the disease even though there are some atypical features, such as seizures or lack of coordination early in the course of disease or other potentially dementing conditions, such as stroke. *Probable Alzheimer's disease* describes dementia with a typical gradual onset and progressive development and *without* any other potentially dementing systemic or brain disorder. *Definite Alzheimer's disease* applies only when clinical diagnosis has been confirmed by evaluation of brain tissue at autopsy, with the tissue showing neuritic plaques and neurofibrillary tangles—the two major hallmarks of Alzheimer's disease as characterized by Alzheimer himself. There is some controversy over *how many* plaques and tangles are required to warrant a diagnosis of definite Alzheimer's disease. In most situations, the issue is not important; someone who had the symptoms of the disease in life and is shown to have any neuritic plaques and neurofibrillary tangles is said to have had definite Alzheimer's disease.

The question of how many plaques and tangles are present becomes more important, however, when a pathologist with no knowledge of the cognitive status of the patient examines a brain. As a result, various diagnostic criteria have been proposed with cut-offs for numbers of plaques and/or tangles, and Alzheimer's disease is diagnosed only when a certain number is present. Though this is not entirely consistent with current understanding of the progression of the disease, it is done for practical purposes. The most frequently cited criteria for this purpose were developed by the National Institute on Aging. They are based on the number of plaques per square millimeter (about 0.00155 square inch) in one area of the brain, and vary according to the age of the patient. Plaque type is not specified. The criteria have been of some use but have been criticized because they cause overdiagnosis of Alzheimer's disease by allowing, for example, nondemented elderly with large numbers of *diffuse plaques* (a type of plaque seen in both normal elderly people and people with Alzheimer's) to qualify as having the disease. A second set of criteria, published by the Consortium to Establish a Registry for Alzheimer's Disease (CERAD), specifies a certain number of neuritic plaques (the type of plaque most commonly seen in Alzheimer's disease) correlated with age and also figures in the presence or absence of Alzheimer's disease symptoms in life, where possible.

In any case, studies comparing the diagnosis made according to the NINCDS-ADRDA criteria while someone is living to the diagnosis made later at autopsy have shown that clinical diagnoses of Alzheimer's disease are correct 80 to 90 percent of the time. Another frequently used set of criteria can be found in the DSM-IV—the Diagnostic and Statistical Manual of Mental Disorders, 4th Edition, published by the

American Psychiatric Association. Here dementia is defined as progressive loss of intellectual capacity severe enough to interfere with everyday activity and with social and interpersonal relationships. This set of criteria is compatible with NINCDS-ADRDA, as can be seen in appendix A.

In order to use these or any other criteria, a physician needs to collect enormous amounts of information. People who come to the doctor with suspected Alzheimer's disease will go through a variety of procedures that enable doctors to determine the cause of the problems as well as possible. We will discuss these procedures in detail.

MEDICAL HISTORY

A careful medical history is the most critical part of the initial evaluation. In addition to talking to the patient, the physician will want to question a family member or close friend, since people with Alzheimer's disease may be unaware of their own deficits. During the history, the physician will inquire about the person's most troublesome symptoms and try to determine how much these have affected daily activities. The physician will ask a number of questions, such as: Can you take care of your personal needs? What about your household and financial responsibilities? Do you have difficulty driving? Do you become easily lost or disoriented? Have you been unusually irritable lately?

The physician will also try to clarify the mode of onset, progression, and duration of the symptoms. Alzheimer's disease evolves gradually over many months and years. There may be patterns that suggest other underlying disorders. If symptoms develop over days or weeks, for example, then depression, a central nervous system infection, or a brain tumor are all reasonable suspicions. A clouded consciousness might suggest an underlying infection or metabolic or toxic problems. Deterioration that has progressed in steps, with periods of sudden deterioration followed by plateaus or even some improvement, suggests multi-infarct dementia, especially if the patient has had a history of high blood pressure or other vascular disease. Other signs of multi-infarct dementia not usually associated with Alzheimer's disease that might be noted at the first medical history include mild paralysis of one side of the body and an abnormal walking pattern.

In order to exclude depression, since severe depression can mimic dementia, the physician will ask about any unusual sleep patterns or weight loss and signs of sadness or pessimism. Depressed people frequently speak freely about their memory lapses, which cause them great distress, whereas Alzheimer's patients are more likely to be unaware of their memory lapses or to hide them when they are aware. If depression is contributing to someone's mental decline, the depression can be treated and any remaining impairment can be evaluated later on.

The medical history should also include an analysis of any drugs being taken by the person that might cause cognitive defects or otherwise affect the central nervous system. These may include prescription medications such as digitalis (for heart problems), insulin (for diabetes), some ulcer medications, high blood pressure medications, narcotic-based painkillers (e.g., codeine-containing drugs, morphine, Demerol®, Darvon®), and a variety of psychiatric medications (e.g., Thorazine®, Valium®). Don't overlook the possible influence of over-the-counter medications, including non-steroidal anti-inflammatory agents (e.g., aspirin or ibuprofen), steroids, cold and allergy medications (e.g., Benadryl®, Sudafed®), and diuretics. Since elderly people often take a number of medications simultaneously, drug interactions are especially important to consider.

The history should also include questions about any history of other medical diseases, trauma, surgery, psychiatric disorders, alcohol intake, nutrition, or exposure to environmental toxins, as well as family history of dementia, Down syndrome, or psychiatric conditions.

PHYSICAL AND NEUROLOGICAL EXAMINATION

The same physician will generally then perform a thorough physical and neurological examination. The diagnosis of Alzheimer's disease requires excluding a wide spectrum of vascular, infectious, and metabolic disorders, including multi-infarct dementia, Parkinson's disease, brain tumor, thyroid disease, HIV, and neurosyphilis and other central nervous system infections. Dementia may also be caused if toxins build up in the brain because of kidney or liver disease (renal or hepatic encephalopathy), or if blood levels of oxygen or carbon dioxide are too low or too high, respectively, both of which conditions can be caused by certain lung diseases.

The physician will perform a series of sensory and motor skills tests, which in the early stages of Alzheimer's disease should be largely normal. Specific signs associated with other potentially dementing conditions include tremors, stiffness, and slowing of movement in Parkinson's disease, muscle spasms and stiffness in Creutzfeldt-Jakob disease, writhing movements in Huntington's disease, abnormal walking in multi-infarct dementia, and difficulties with walking in normal pressure hydrocephalus.

Patients should be given a chest X-ray to rule out lung diseases and an electrocardiogram to rule out the presence of ischemic heart disease, which may result in cerebral ischemia (a reduction in blood flow to the brain) and cause dementia. Laboratory urine and blood tests will help in identifying or eliminating metabolic or nutritional conditions and diseases of the liver, kidney, and thyroid. A spinal tap may be done to allow the analysis of cerebrospinal fluid, a fluid found in the brain and spinal cord, in order to detect any chronic infection. An electroencephalogram (EEG), a measure of the electrical activity of the brain, can be performed as well. In the early stages of Alzheimer's disease, the EEG is normal, but later on changes are seen in up to 90 percent of patients, so an abnormal EEG may indicate later-stage disease. EEGs can also help physicians to detect and rule out certain seizure disorders in which subtle seizures that are undetectable to observers cause a confused state resembling dementia.

MENTAL STATUS TESTING

Mental status testing is used to help the physician determine the extent of cognitive and behavioral impairment. The patient is asked to answer questions and/or perform various tasks. Questions might include "What is the date today?" and "Who is the president of the United States?" Tasks to be performed could include drawing a clock face on an empty circle, putting paper in an envelope and indicating where the stamp goes, counting backwards by 7s from 100, naming objects shown in pictures, or reciting words given several minutes back. At the completion of a mental status test, a numerical score is assigned that can be compared to average values determined in larger groups of people at varying levels of impairment. This allows the doctor to see where the patient falls in the spectrum of possible scores and to get an idea of the severity of the impairment.

Different tests have been designed to assess dementia and Alzheimer's characteristics in general, measure the severity of disease, rate the patient's functional impairment (i.e., how well the patient functions in everyday life), and assess noncognitive behavioral symptoms. Some of the more common tests a doctor might use are the Mini-Mental State Examination, the Blessed Dementia Rating Scale, and the Mattis Dementia Rating Scale. Although the Mini-Mental is widely used to identify deficits in orientation and memory as well as in verbal, numerical, and spatial ability, it may falsely signal dementia in poorly educated but normal people or permit mildly demented people to appear normal. Neuropsychological testing is an inexact science, and, in all tests, cut-off points designed to separate normal from demented people should be used in the context of an individual's history and condition. This is especially true regarding Alzheimer's disease, since patients exhibit a wide spectrum of cognitive and behavioral deficits that may differ from person to person, making it extremely difficult for the scores on any one neuropsychological test to point reliably to the diagnosis. Social, cultural, and educational factors should also be considered in evaluations of neuropsychological test results.

Even with their various drawbacks, neuropsychological evaluations are helpful in determining the deficits of a particular person, and can aid in developing an appropriate management plan later on and ruling out other conditions. For example, the NINCDS-ADRDA Work Group recommends use of the Hamilton Rating Scale for Depression to evaluate the severity of depression, the Present State Examination for anxiety, depression, delusions, and hallucinations, and the Hachinski Ischemia Scale to evaluate the possibility of strokes and multi-infarct dementia.

BRAIN SCANS

Brain scans (neuroimaging) provide images of the brain's structures. Computed tomography (CT) scanning, sometimes called computerized axial tomography (CAT), or magnetic resonance imaging (MRI) should be a routine step in the diagnostic work-up of someone with symptoms of dementia. CT scanning passes X-rays through the brain; then computers analyze the changes in the X-rays to put together images of slices of the brain. MRI works much the same way, using magnetic beams instead of X-rays. Hydrogen atoms in the brain, mostly in the form of water (H_2O), emit electromagnetic waves that change their patterns when magnetic beams pass through them. Because the quantity of water in gray and white matter (two types of brain tissue) and brain fluid varies, computers hooked up to special magnetic detectors can differentiate among the different brain tissues to create a visual representation of the brain.

MRI is a bit more flexible than CT scanning because it can create images along three different planes of the brain, whereas CT can create images along only one. CT scanning has the advantage, however, of being widely available, familiar to physicians and patients, and more comfortable for patients since it is faster and less noisy and claustrophobia-inducing than MRI. Recent technology has further increased the speed of CT scanning, which is particularly helpful when imaging Alzheimer's disease patients, who may become distressed or have difficulty remaining motionless for the length of time required.

Neither of these procedures can diagnose Alzheimer's disease absolutely, but both are useful for ruling out certain anatomically caused conditions. The CT scan can detect such potentially treatable conditions as brain tumors, blood clots, hydrocephalus, and damaged blood vessels, which do not always produce obvious symptoms and are therefore easily confused with other dementing disorders. In people with Alzheimer's disease, CT scans may show evidence of cerebral atrophy, and there is evidence that such atrophy is on average greater in the brains of Alzheimer's patients than in normal controls (figs. 1.1a and 1.1b). Evidence of atrophy does not define Alzheimer's disease, however, because there is considerable overlap in the ranges of atrophy for normal people and Alzheimer's patients, and because such atrophy is often seen in other dementias.

MRI allows the visual characterization of anomalies even in the very small brain structures that may be affected in Alzheimer's disease. Although it is similar to CT scanning in its ability to detect gross anatomical defects, MRI is better able to detect the smaller infarcts common in multi-infarct dementia. Though some studies have found that MRI results in overdiagnosis of multi-infarct dementia because certain irrelevant white matter structures closely resemble infarcts,

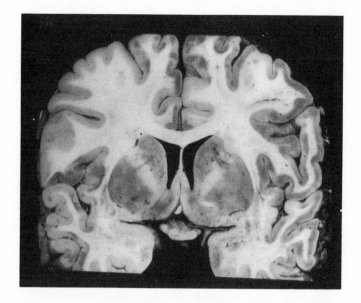

FIG 1.1a. Autopsy cross-sections of a normal elderly brain (a) and a brain affected by Alzheimer's disease (b). Notice the deterioration of the solid part of the brain in (b). Figure from Cutler NR, Sramek JJ, Veroff AE. *Alzheimer's Disease: Optimizing Drug Development Strategies,* © 1994, John Wiley & Sons, Ltd. Reprinted by permission.

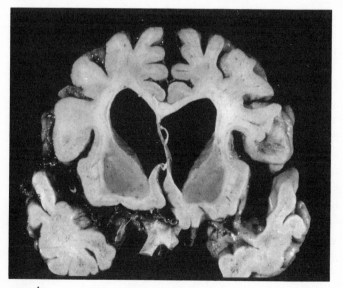

FIG 1.1b.

the technique shows great promise for distinguishing between multi-infarct dementia and Alzheimer's disease.

Positron emission tomography (PET) and single-photon emission computed tomography (SPECT) are two other imaging techniques, both more expensive and less widely available than CT and MRI. Rather than allowing visualization of tissue substance and anatomy, as do CT and MRI, these two techniques permit investigators to see which parts of the brain are working the hardest during particular mental activities. First, a slightly radioactive form of the sugar glucose is injected into a person's bloodstream. Since glucose is the form of energy used by the brain, glucose will travel to all brain cells that are using energy—in other words, the active ones. Radiation detectors can track the movement of the glucose to produce a picture of the brain's activity. Because different parts of the brain show activity depending on what the subject is doing, or even what the subject is thinking about, PET and SPECT scans are far more complicated than CT or MRI scans. Researchers must collect more information about the images produced with these methods by normal brains before they can be used for diagnosing abnormal brains. Though at this time PET or SPECT remain primarily research tools, there is reason to believe that they may become more useful for diagnosis in the future.

Families often worry about what to tell someone who has been diagnosed with Alzheimer's disease. Physicians generally agree that it is best to be honest and let people know what is causing their problems. Most people are relieved to know that they are not going "crazy," and that there is a cause for whatever symptoms they may be experiencing. Furthermore, this keeps the lines of communication between patients and families open and allows the person to participate as fully as possible in planning for the future.

Initially Alzheimer's patients and their families may deal with only one doctor—a family doctor, perhaps, or a geriatrician, neurologist, or psychiatrist. Eventually, however, complete care may involve the advice and expertise of a variety of professionals, including lawyers, accountants, social workers, nurses, counselors, physical therapists, and clergy. The various aspects of patient care will be discussed in greater depth in chapter 4.

2. The Brain

Many interrelated events in the brains of people with Alzheimer's disease lead to the symptoms we associate with it. A basic understanding of how the brain works will permit a better understanding of these events and how they cause Alzheimer's disease. The brain contains approximately 100 billion nerve cells, or *neurons*, which are its working components. They control our muscles, contain our memories, receive sensory information, cause hormones to be produced, and control our emotions.

Neurons are composed of several parts (fig. 2.1). Long thin projections called *dendrites* branch out from the central cell body and bring impulses to the neuron. Another long thin strand, the *axon*, projects out and sends impulses to other cells. Axons range in length from a tiny fraction of an inch, when they extend only to a neighboring neuron, to several feet, when they extend to cells in other parts of the body. Both axons and dendrites are *neurites*, a word used to describe any cylindrical extension of a neuron. As we shall see, abnormalities in neurites of both types are present in Alzheimer's disease.

Communication between neurons is achieved when chemicals called *neurotransmitters* move from one neuron to another. For example, an important neurotransmitter relevant to Alzheimer's disease is *acetylcholine*, which is found in around 15 percent of the brain's neurons, or about 15 billion of them. Acetylcholine is stored inside the neuron in small pockets near the surface of an axon. Axons come very close to but do not touch the dendrites of neighboring neurons at junctions called *synapses*. The gap between the adjacent synapses of two neurons is called the *synaptic cleft*. The neuron sending a message discharges acetylcholine molecules into

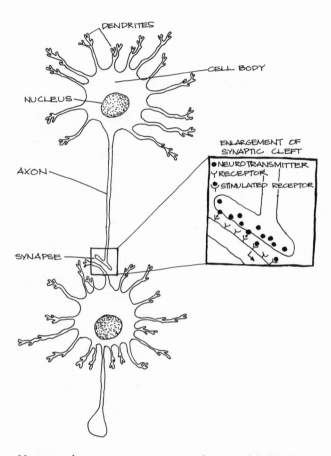

FIG 2.1. Neurons release neurotransmitters such as acetylcholine from their axons. The neurotransmitters travel across the synapse and attach to the next cell on specialized molecules called receptors, each designed to recognize particular neurotransmitters.

the synaptic cleft, where they briefly attach to special proteins, called *receptors*, on the surface of a dendrite. When enough receptors are stimulated, the receiving neuron responds to the message by sending an electrical impulse down the length of its axon until it reaches the axon terminal, where its own neurotransmitters will be released to stimulate receptors on the next neuron. This is how the message is transmitted. Meanwhile, the acetylcholine that was released into the synaptic cleft is deactivated by an enzyme called *acetylcholinesterase* and then reabsorbed by the transmitting neuron to be used again. Deactivating acetylcholine is important because if left in the system for too long, it could overstimulate neurons in certain organs and result in disastrous consequences, such as an inability to move or breathe.

Each of the brain's billions of neurons is directly or indirectly connected to every other. There are also many different neurotransmitters that may be released alone or in combination to make up different kinds of messages. Each neuron has numerous synapses, so a given neuron might receive messages from up to several hundred neurons and send messages to a like number. Activation of some receptors stimulates a neuron to send a message; activation of other receptors inhibits the sending of a message.

Throughout life, people lose neurons, perhaps up to 100,000 neurons per day after reaching age 30—which adds up to 2 billion cells over 50 years. While this sounds like a large number, 2 billion is only 2 percent of the brain's estimated 100 billion cells. Furthermore, most bodily organs have more than enough cells to do their job, and many neurologists believe the brain does, too. While neurons can never be replaced, the brain appears to have two mechanisms for dealing with the destruction of neurons (fig. 2.2). One protection is *redundancy*: many neurons perform identical functions, and a given message can be sent along any of a large number of neurons. If a few are destroyed, there are often other neurons that can relay the same message just as well. Neurons can also sprout new connections and in doing so repair or compensate for

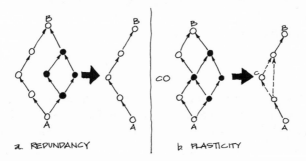

FIG 2.2. Schematic diagram of neural connections. Circles represent neurons, and arrows represent the connections between neurons, showing
the pathways along which messages can be sent. (a) Redundancy: If the
four shaded neurons are destroyed, a message can still get from neuron
A to neuron B. (b) Plasticity: If the original connections do not include
neuron C, and the four shaded neurons are destroyed, a new pathway
or new pathways may form along the dotted lines.

broken circuits that result when a neuron dies. The capacity
of the brain to adapt in this manner is referred to as *plasticity*.

Learning, in fact, is a process of making new connections
between neurons in the brain. The more you learn, the more
connected your neurons become. Major intellectual functions
are dependent on this interconnectedness. The ability to
retain use of these functions depends, then, on the structural
stability of individual neurons and their synapses as well as
their connections to each other.

3. What Causes Alzheimer's Disease?

Over the past century there has been a variety of explanations for Alzheimer's disease. Some have been largely discounted, while many others are still being investigated. It seems likely that the symptoms of Alzheimer's disease are the result of several processes in the brain, and determining how these processes fit together and in what order they occur is a great challenge. Furthermore, evidence suggests that there may be more than one form of the disease, each with its own prevalent features. We will present a few theories about the causes of Alzheimer's disease that have been popular in the past, explaining why they are no longer in favor, and then we will go into current theories in greater detail.

LARGELY DISCOUNTED THEORIES

At one time, Alzheimer's disease was thought to be caused by strokes and build-up of foreign substances in the blood vessels of the brain. Neuroimaging techniques that enable physicians to actually see various parts of a living person's brain have demonstrated that strokes are not a large risk factor for Alzheimer's disease, and, instead, that such strokes lead to a separate type of dementia known as multiple-infarct dementia (see chapter 1). Some people have both disorders at the same time, but they are distinct entities. The majority of people with Alzheimer's disease do not suffer from strokes.

Another largely discounted theory is that Alzheimer's disease is caused by a virus. Most viruses, such as those that cause the common cold or measles, make their hosts sick within a few days after infection, and the infection clears up once the person's immune system has a chance to destroy the virus. A different type of virus called a "slow virus," however, is able to lie dormant in its host for years before causing any kind of illness. Shingles and AIDS, for example, are illnesses that occur years after the initial viral infection. The theory that Alzheimer's disease might involve the actions of a slow virus came about because certain other rare dementias, including Creutzfeldt-Jakob disease, *Gerstmann-Straussler syndrome*, and *kuru*, are caused by unusual, slow-acting viruses. There is no good evidence, however, to show that this is so. While studying slow viruses may provide some insight into some types of dementias, most experts agree that such studies will not help us to find the cause behind Alzheimer's disease.

Many researchers have hunted for evidence that Alzheimer's is caused by various substances in the environment or in our bodies that have the potential to act as toxins (poisons). Many substances are toxic only in large quantities. For example, the body requires small amounts of iodine—most of which we get from ingesting iodized salt—but too much iodine would be poisonous and result in the need for medical treatment. The best-known environmental substance studied in connection with Alzheimer's disease is aluminum. We all have some aluminum in our bodies, which is generally nothing to worry about. Aluminum levels increase dramatically in people who undergo kidney dialysis regularly, because the process of dialysis involves aluminum, and some of these people suffer from dementia symptoms in what is known as aluminum intoxication. Though this dementia is reversible after treatment to remove the excess aluminum, the association of aluminum with dementia in patients on kidney dialysis led to investigations of aluminum's potential role in Alzheimer's disease.

Several researchers have found elevated levels of aluminum in Alzheimer's patients in areas of the brain affected by the disease. The excess is extremely small, however, and it is yet to be determined whether or not excesses of aluminum are common to all aged brains. The biological function of aluminum, if any, is unknown. It may participate in chemical reactions, but this seems unlikely. Scientists know that if they inject aluminum into the brains of laboratory animals, the animals will develop brain lesions similar to neurofibrillary tangles. However, animals with aluminum-related lesions do not display any behaviors that could be considered the animal equivalent of dementia, so it is difficult to say what the presence of aluminum actually means. It could be that when neurons die, any aluminum that was in them moves to other neurons, so that people with Alzheimer's disease have more highly concentrated levels of aluminum in their neurons. In this case, the presence of aluminum might be completely irrelevant to the development of Alzheimer's disease. Alternatively, aluminum *might* be responsible for killing nerve cells and remain there after nerve cell death.

In any case, our technological society constantly exposes us to aluminum. The likely explanation for a slight excess of aluminum is that there is some fault in the person's metabolic processing of the substance. The chances are good that exposure to aluminum is completely unrelated to the mental decline and behavioral problems that come with Alzheimer's disease. Most people who have Alzheimer's were not exposed to high levels of aluminum, and most people with high exposure do not develop the disease.

CURRENT THEORIES

Genetics

A major question for researchers concerns whether or not Alzheimer's disease is hereditary. A brief review of the basics of genetics may be helpful in understanding the relationship between it and Alzheimer's disease. Genes are the blueprints of the body. They carry all the information needed for life in coded form on long strands of a chemical called

DNA. The chemical codes embedded in the DNA are read by cells, and serve to control the production of proteins—from determining which proteins should be made by which cells to regulating when they start and stop. Many proteins start out relatively large but are later cut into parts. Some large proteins become several smaller useful proteins, while others become just one smaller protein along with some waste material. This refinement process is known as the *metabolism* of the protein, or, less formally, as the *processing* of the protein, and it is controlled by the same gene that codes for the protein.

Proteins serve many functions. Some serve as building materials and last a long time. Others become enzymes, the molecules that allow chemical reactions to happen in our bodies, and may be needed for only a short time. When a protein is no longer needed, it is usually transported to an area of the cell where enzymes cut the protein up into little bits. The building blocks that were used to make the protein can then be taken elsewhere to make other proteins. The breaking down of a protein that is no longer needed is known as "digestion." Because some proteins are meant to last and others are not, some proteins are easily digested, while others are completely indigestible.

Through DNA, our genes control every aspect of our growth and development and allow us to function as human beings. All genes come in pairs, and are stored in groups on paired *chromosomes*, larger structures that help to organize the genes within the control center of a cell, the nucleus. Every cell except for red blood cells and *gametes* (egg cells and sperm cells) has a complete set of chromosomes—46 in all, neatly organized into 23 pairs. The gametes have only 23 chromosomes each, so that when they meet at conception, the chromosomes join up to make 23 matching pairs in the new, rapidly dividing cells that will grow to become a person. All people, then, are born with 23 chromosomes from their mother and 23 from their father. When one reads of a defect on, say, "chromosome 14," what is meant is a defect on a gene on one or both of the chromosomes that make up the 14th chromosome *pair*. On each matched pair of chromosomes there are series of genes that also match up. One half of a gene pair—that is, a gene on just one chromosome—is called an *allele*, and it works in concert with another allele, the matching gene on the chromosome paired with its own. All physical characteristics are controlled by at least one of these allele pairs.

Investigation of the relationship between Alzheimer's disease and genetics has provided substantial evidence that there are several forms of Alzheimer's disease. A small percentage of Alzheimer's disease cases tends to run in families and is known as *familial Alzheimer's disease*. The majority of cases, called *sporadic Alzheimer's disease*, do not run in families. It seems likely that all types have at least some hereditary component, but the extent to which genetics influences someone's risk of developing the disease depends on the type of Alzheimer's disease.

A gene can be linked to a disease in two different ways: it can cause the disease or it can be a factor contributing to the risk of developing the disease. In the first case, a person with one or more defective genes invariably contracts the disease—the progression of the disease is programmed by that person's genes. Although the disease may not appear for many years, the approximate time of its arrival can be predicted, just as the changes of puberty can be predicted once a person's sex is known. A genetically programmed disease may be the result of one gene, just as the presence of absence of hair on the middle joint of a person's fingers is determined by one gene, or it can result from several genes, in the same way that several genes contribute to eye color. Usually, however, the hereditary factor in a disease is not strong enough to make the disease a foregone conclusion. Genes can contribute to the risk of getting a disease without necessarily causing the disease. For example, it is well known that obesity is a risk factor for heart disease. Some types of obesity are hereditary, so a person who is predisposed to being overweight would also have a higher risk of heart disease. Not every obese person develops heart disease, however. A person with a gene for obesity may or may not develop heart disease, because the gene does not directly cause heart disease. The gene only increases the susceptibility to heart disease. This kind of increased susceptibility to a disease is called a genetic factor. Health behaviors can influence the likelihood of one's developing a disease that has a genetic factor. For example, a nonsmoker with a gene for obesity who exercises regularly and eats a low-salt, low-fat, healthy diet is less likely to develop heart disease than a smoker with the same gene who never exercises and does not eat well.

How can researchers tell if a disease is entirely determined by the genes, has a genetic factor, or is unrelated to heredity? Identical twins can provide a clue, because they have exactly the same genes. When a disease is entirely genetic, if one twin has it, the other will have it too, regardless of environmental factors. If the disease is unrelated to heredity, then the second twin should have no more chance of getting the disease than anybody else raised in the same environment. If there is a genetic factor, then the second identical twin should be more likely than other people to contract the disease, but the incidence should be somewhere between 40 and 60 percent—far below the nearly 100 percent seen in purely genetic diseases. The existence of a genetic risk factor can be established based on the incidence of the disease in families even before the exact nature of the risk factor is determined.

Familial Alzheimer's disease, which probably represents no more than 10 percent of all Alzheimer's cases, is a purely genetic disease caused by a single defective gene. Sporadic Alzheimer's disease, on the other hand, has a genetic risk factor and perhaps environmental risk factors, too. In general, the risk of developing any type of Alzheimer's disease is three to four times greater if a close relative has the disease, but it is important to keep this risk factor in perspective.

While approximately 25 percent to 30 percent of people with
Alzheimer's disease have another demented relative, 70 percent to 75 percent of Alzheimer's patients *do not* have another
demented relative. Some people believe that the hereditary
component of Alzheimer's disease would appear more impres-
sive if there were a way for investigators to find out whether
family members who died before reaching the higher risk
years for Alzheimer's disease would have developed it.

In familial Alzheimer's disease, the children of an Alzheimer's
patient have a 50–50 chance of also developing dementia.
If both parents have it, this chance increases to 75 percent.
Every generation is affected, men and women are equally
likely to develop the disease, and environmental factors have

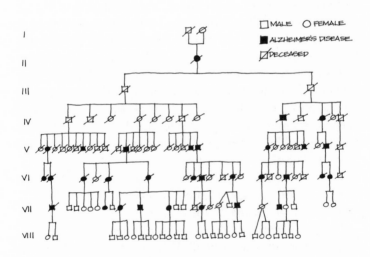

FIG 3.1. Pedigree of family with familial Alzheimer's disease. Some not
diagnosed with Alzheimer's may have died before the disease could
be noticed, some may have had it but no medical records or family
memories show this, and some probably did not have it. Members of
the youngest generation are all represented by empty shapes because
they are still too young to have expressed the disease, though all are
at risk.

little apparent influence (fig. 3.1). For affected people in many of these families, the illness strikes at a young age—the 40s or 50s. It is clear from these cases that familial Alzheimer's disease is genetically programmed. These large families with multigenerational (and frequently early-onset) Alzheimer's disease, however, probably represent no more than 10 percent of all Alzheimer's patients. Most people, even those with a history of dementia in their family, do not appear to be at risk for Alzheimer's disease to the extent that members of these families are.

At one time, age of onset was thought to be a good indicator of whether or not a given case of Alzheimer's disease is familial. Because several commonly studied families with familial Alzheimer's disease showed consistent early onset of disease, scientists hypothesized that early onset was a sign of familial Alzheimer's disease. Even though early onset *is* more common among familial types of the disease than in sporadic Alzheimer's disease, late onset is more common than early onset in both sporadic and familial types. One problem with analyses based on age is that there is no consensus regarding what constitutes early versus late onset. Most agree that before 50 or 55 is early and after 70 is late, but the cut-off in between is more arbitrary, though frequently set at age 65. It appears that even within familial Alzheimer's disease, the illness can be classified according to age of onset and various other features. Survival time after diagnosis seems relatively consistent regardless of age of onset.

The search for genetic causes for either type of Alzheimer's disease began when physicians noticed that nearly all people with Down syndrome who live into their late 30s develop brain degeneration remarkably similar to that seen in Alzheimer's. This similarity spurred scientists to look for a genetic defect in Alzheimer's disease patients on chromosome 21, the chromosome related to Down syndrome. Sure enough, scientists found a problem with one gene on chromosome 21 in about 5 percent of the families with early-onset familial

Alzheimer's disease. The defective gene is responsible for the production of amyloid precursor protein (APP), a large protein that is normally involved in cell growth and repair. After leaving the cell where it is produced, part of the protein is cut off and made into a smaller protein. Usually it is cut up to become soluble-APP (s-APP), a protein that is easily digested by the body when it is no longer needed. Less often it is cut up to become beta amyloid, a small, indigestible protein that tends to accumulate in plaques. The accumulation of too much beta amyloid can cause problems, as we shall see below. The defects in the APP gene seen in affected families alter the processing of the protein in some way that leads to Alzheimer's disease, most likely by increasing production of beta amyloid. Scientists have discovered that abnormal processing of APP can be caused not just by defects in the processing of APP, but by any excess of APP. This helps to explain what might happen in Down syndrome patients, who produce more APP than normal, because they carry an extra copy of chromosome 21.

In any case, defects in chromosome 21 are present in fewer than 1 percent of Alzheimer's disease patients. Most of these patients develop the illness early in their lives, usually before age 65. Thus these defects are responsible for only one type of Alzheimer's disease. Most people with familial Alzheimer's disease develop the disease after age 65, and further, 90 percent of people who have Alzheimer's do not even have familial Alzheimer's disease. Thus the genetic defect on chromosome 21 accounts for only some cases of Alzheimer's disease. Researchers have expanded their search for genetic causes of this disease; what they have found is summarized in table 3.1.

There appear to be four major strains of familial Alzheimer's disease, three of which show early onset. One of these involves the previously discussed defect in the APP gene on chromosome 21. In the summer of 1995, the other two early-onset strains were found to be associated with defects in two very similar genes located on chromosomes 1 and 14. One of

Table 3.1. Genes that have been associated with Alzheimer's disease

Type of Alzheimer's disease	Associated chromosome	Product of affected gene
Familial		
early onset	21	amyloid precursor protein (APP)
early onset	14	S182 (membrane protein)
early onset	1	STM2 (membrane protein)
late onset	19	apolipoprotein E (apoE)
Sporadic		
early onset	19	apoE
late onset	19	apoE

them, S182, appears to be responsible for 70–80 percent of all early-onset familial Alzheimer's disease (5–10 percent of all Alzheimer's disease), and the other, STM2, is responsible for perhaps 20 percent of familial cases (2–3 percent of all cases).[2] While the exact function of these genes is unknown, both are involved in the production of proteins embedded in membranes, possibly controlling what can go in and out of cellular compartments.

There is much speculation about how alterations in these two genes might cause Alzheimer's disease, but nothing is known for sure yet. An early guess came from evidence that patients with a defect in the S182 gene make abnormally high amounts of beta amyloid—the same protein whose overabundance is implicated in patients with defects in the APP gene on chromosome 21. Researchers theorized that perhaps the mutations in S182 and STM2 change the ability of cells to transport APP, permitting the protein to stay too long in conditions that promote the formation of beta amyloid or not long enough in conditions that prevent it. What these conditions might be is yet unknown. A more recent guess comes from the early 1996 finding that STM2 appears to be the human version of a mouse gene found to be involved in the control of *programmed cell death*, a natural process in which old cells are methodically destroyed to make room for new ones. Abnormalities in this process contribute to many diseases, including cancer and AIDS, and could very well contribute to Alzheimer's disease. At this point, all we know is that parts of STM2 are nearly identical to a mouse gene that is involved in regulating programmed cell death in mice. If scientists can show that STM2 is indeed involved in regulating this process *in humans*, this would suggest that the genetic mutation seen in STM2 in some people with familial Alzheimer's disease is disrupting the process, leading to un-controlled and premature death of neurons—and eventually to Alzheimer's disease. And if STM2 and S182 are closely related, this could also explain the Alzheimer's disease of patients with mutations on the S182 gene.

The coming years will undoubtedly shed light on the nor-mal functions of S182 and STM2, the proteins they code for, and their relationship to programmed cell death. Ultimately we may definitively know how these genes contribute to the development of Alzheimer's disease. There might be an entire previously unknown family of proteins similar to S182 and STM2, and they may all have similar functions. Some might even be involved in the 90 percent of Alzheimer's cases that are not familial. This could mean that other, as yet undiscov-ered, proteins have a hand in causing sporadic Alzheimer's disease. And, though no one is sure yet, programmed cell death might have something to do with it.

Studies of the set of families who have late-onset famil-ial Alzheimer's disease show a link between the illness and a gene on chromosome 19. Research on possible genetic influences in this collection of families has been considered extremely important because late onset is typical of the more common, sporadic form of the disease. The specific target gene on chromosome 19 is thought to be the APO E gene, which codes for *apolipoprotein E*, a protein that is involved in movement of cholesterol in and out of cells throughout the body. There are three slightly different forms of the gene— APO E2, APO E3, and APO E4. Everyone has two copies of the APO E gene, one from each parent. They may have any combination of the different types of APO E genes—two APO E2 genes, for example, or one APO E3 and one APO E4, and so on. The presence of the APO E4 form greatly increases one's risk for late-onset familial Alzheimer's disease. Perhaps the most dramatic finding regarding the APO E gene came later, however, when it was shown that APO E4 is a major risk factor for Alzheimer's disease in general, regardless of age at onset or family history. An individual with two copies of APO E4 has a risk of developing Alzheimer's disease fifteen times greater than someone with no copies of APO E4, and someone with one copy of APO E4 has five times the risk. It also appears that the APO E2 form decreases the risk of the disease and increases the age of onset of the disease when it does occur. One study showed that people who inherit both an APO E2 and an APO E3 gene develop Alzheimer's on average 20 years later than those who inherit two APO E4 genes.

Recent studies have bolstered the strength of these findings. A study published in 1995 analyzed the PET scans of 38 people over 40 who either had Alzheimer's disease or were related to someone with Alzheimer's disease.[3] Relatives of Alzheimer's patients showed no signs of the disease and were divided into two groups: those with one or two copies of the APO E4 gene and those with no copies of the APO E4 gene. In the people with Alzheimer's disease, PET scans showed a decrease of brain activity in the areas where thought processes are concentrated, as compared to normal subjects. Relatives with one or two APO E4 genes showed the same types of decreases in brain activity, but the deviations from normal were less severe. Relatives with no APO E4 genes had normal PET scans. These results suggest that the subtle changes in the brain that lead to Alzheimer's disease begin long before the disease is noticed. Also, it seems that perhaps there is no particular defect in a gene on chromosome 19 causing Alzheimer's disease (as there are for the genes on chromosomes 1, 14, and 21), but that the presence of a particular form of a gene contributes to the development of the disease. Much of the current research on the causes of Alzheimer's disease centers around the role of the APO E gene and its product, apolipoprotein E, and we will discuss some of the more recent findings below.

Except for a few families with defects in chromosomes 1, 14, and 21, genetic defects are not the major cause of Alzheimer's disease. It does appear that the APO E gene, particularly the presence or absence of the APO E4 form of the gene, plays a role in perhaps 50 percent of disease cases, but even so, not everyone who carries APO E4 develops the disease, and not everyone with Alzheimer's disease carries APO E4. Clearly, multiple factors are at work.[4] In the next sections we will focus on the structural and biochemical changes that occur in the brains of people who have Alzheimer's disease in order to sort out what happens.

CHANGES IN THE BRAIN

What actually causes signs of dementia in people with Alzheimer's disease? Perhaps the most significant direct cause of dementia is a loss of neurons. Neuropathologists (scientists who study abnormalities of the brain) note a major loss of large neurons in areas of the brain associated with higher mental functions. As mentioned earlier, neuron death is a normal part of aging, but somehow neurons die faster in people with Alzheimer's disease than in other people. A great enough loss of neurons will interfere with normal mental functioning.

At first, people can compensate by using alternate neurons—there are so many, after all, that losing a few is generally not a problem. But as the loss becomes greater, mental functioning is bound to suffer. At some critical point, the brain is no longer able to compensate for the loss, and symptoms begin to appear.

When we refer to neuron loss, we are not necessarily referring to the complete *death* of a neuron, but rather to the loss of its functioning. Neuron functions may shut down some time before a neuron actually dies, and some neurons may even regain functioning if the damage is not too severe. Scientists measure neuron loss indirectly, by measuring chemicals that are used and/or produced when neurons function normally.

For example, the activity of an enzyme called *choline acetyltransferase*, required for the production of the neurotransmitter acetylcholine, is greatly reduced in the brain tissue of those with Alzheimer's disease, probably as a result of damage to and/or loss of neurons. The reduction of activity causes a decrease in acetylcholine production, which then hinders normal communication between neurons and leads to deficits in brain function. As we shall see in chapter 6, correction of the acetylcholine deficit as well as other neurotransmitter deficits is currently thought to be a promising route to alleviating some of the cognitive symptoms of Alzheimer's disease.

Another factor affecting neuron functioning is synapse loss. The normal firing of a neuron usually requires stimulation of many receptors, often at more than one synapse. If one neuron stops working, it will stop stimulating connected neurons, making all their shared synapses useless. If enough synapses are lost, even undamaged neurons may not receive enough stimulation from the appropriate neurotransmitters to work properly.

Nerve and synapse loss is severe in people with Alzheimer's disease, and this contributes greatly to a reduction of mental functioning. Exactly how neurons and synapses become damaged and lost is not entirely understood, but a number of clues arise from many other changes that occur in the brains of Alzheimer's patients. We will take some time now to describe these changes and explore how they come about.

Physical changes in the brain cannot be seen or felt from the outside without the use of sophisticated equipment. One change that can be detected through use of MRI or CT scans is a reduction in the size of the brain of Alzheimer's patients (see chapter 1). The brain decreases in size somewhat even in normal aging, though, and the reduction in size varies considerably from person to person, making brain size ineffective as a diagnostic tool in the early stages of disease. The most important abnormalities of the diseased brain cannot be detected without microscopic examination of brain tissue at autopsy.

Brain tissue of Alzheimer's patients reveals many abnormal structural changes that affect the workings of the brain. These changes include the appearance of *neuritic plaques* and *neurofibrillary tangles*, which are, as mentioned earlier, the two major "hallmarks" of Alzheimer's disease. These lesions (in medicine, the term "lesion" is used to describe any localized area of injured tissue—such as a wound—or an area where an abnormal structural change has taken place) are both associated with neurons and located in the area of the brain associated with memory, the hippocampus. Because these physical signs of Alzheimer's disease can only be detected at autopsy, it is virtually impossible to determine whether they appear early or late in the course of disease.

A plaque may be thought of as any abnormal deposit of a foreign substance or an unusually large quantity of a natural substance in some kind of body tissue. You may hear Alzheimer's disease-related plaques referred to as "senile plaques" or "amyloid plaques" (amyloid is a substance composed of protein fibers). There are two major types of plaques found in the brains of people with Alzheimer's disease—those involving neurons that still have normal neurites (dendrites and axons) and those involving neurons with damaged neurites. Plaques involving normal neurites are *diffuse plaques.* They generally have cores made up of amyloid with tiny hair-like amyloid wisps coming out of them. Diffuse plaques are found in some normal elderly people and in people who have Alzheimer's disease.

The other major type of plaque, more significant to the Alzheimer's disease process, is the *neuritic plaque* (fig. 3.2). These plaques consist of abnormal neurites—damaged dendrites and axons—surrounding a core of amyloid. They also contain dense arrangements of paired helical filaments. These spiral-shaped structures are made of tau proteins, major structural components of neurons. Other important chemicals frequently associated with plaques include amyloid precursor protein, apolipoprotein E, and many neurotransmitters.

The origin of plaques is poorly understood. According to one hypothesis, neuritic plaques develop from diffuse plaques.

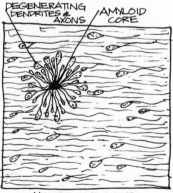

FIG 3.2. A neuritic plaque.

But because there are, in some areas of the brain, diffuse plaques that do not seem ever to change into neuritic plaques, there must be other chemicals or factors that play a role in the areas where neuritic plaques *are* seen.

Abnormal neuritic elements in plaques contain several proteins that are generally associated with synapses and axons. Amyloid precursor protein (APP) is one such molecule. It is likely to be centrally involved in plaque formation. As discussed in the section on genetics, APP is cut up to become one of several varieties of soluble-APP or, less frequently, beta amyloid. In the normal brain, APP is rapidly transported in the axon to the dendrites, and it is also found in growing neurites in fetal brains. Most types of soluble-APP are involved in helping neurons and synapses to grow and maintain integrity. It seems that in Alzheimer's disease, the metabolism of APP is altered so that beta amyloid is formed more often than soluble-APP, instead of the other way around. This causes two associated problems. First, decreased levels of soluble-APP translate to a reduction in the protective effects of this protein, making neurons more susceptible to damage. This sets the stage for beta amyloid, which appears to be able to cause neuron damage both by itself and through jelling in masses as the primary constituent of plaques. No one is quite sure how important these mechanisms are in contributing to the problems seen in Alzheimer's disease, but both may play a role.

Incidentally, Alzheimer's disease is not the only disease that involves amyloid; there are over 16 types of amyloid-associated diseases. Though each type of amyloid has a distinct biochemical form, all share a particular structure and appearance. When any of these fibrous proteins is deposited outside cells, it is known as amyloidosis. Depending on the disease, amyloid deposits may appear almost anywhere—from heart and liver to skin and bone.

The recent discovery that people who carry the APO E4 gene are at higher risk for developing Alzheimer's disease and the presence of apolipoprotein E (apoE) in neuritic plaques has prompted investigation into the role of apoE protein in plaque formation. (Note that "APO E" in capital letters is used to refer to the gene, whereas "apoE" refers to its product, apolipoprotein E.) ApoE normally promotes repair or regeneration of broken connections between neurons. As we have said, beta amyloid causes damage to neurons, so it makes sense that the presence of beta amyloid might spur increased production of apoE in the same areas of the brain. What complicates matters is that apoE binds to beta amyloid easily. When apoE comes into contact with beta amyloid, the two molecules attach to one another, and then apoE is no longer free to help repair the neurons. This allows more neurites to remain damaged—in perfect condition for plaque formation. Furthermore, apoE also appears to work as a kind of glue between molecules of beta amyloid. When apoE is present, beta amyloid is more likely to form deposits that might eventually become plaques. Thus, in binding to beta amyloid, apoE protein actually *helps* plaques to form.

Interestingly, there is some evidence to suggest that people with Alzheimer's who have two copies of the APO E4 gene actually have more neuritic plaques than patients with other gene combinations. The hypothesis that best explains this hinges on the fact that apoE4 protein appears to bind to beta amyloid more strongly and rapidly than the other two forms. This would make apoE4 better than the other two forms at providing glue to form beta amyloid plaques. It also means that the pool of apoE available to protect neurons from the toxic effects of beta amyloid would be reduced to a greater degree with apoE4 than with apoE2 or apoE3. Binding between beta amyloid and apoE does happen for all three types, but it may be that plaque formation is faster for the apoE4 because of its more avid binding.

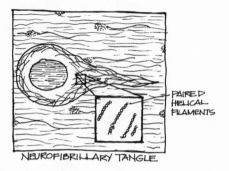

FIG 3.3. A neurofibrillary tangle.

Neurofibrillary tangles are another lesion frequently seen
in those with Alzheimer's disease, though they occur in other
disorders as well. Some older patients, who seem not to have
these tangles, have been sometimes said to have "plaque-only
Alzheimer's disease." Neurofibrillary tangles are made up
largely of paired helical filaments, which are, as mentioned
earlier, made of modified tau proteins (fig. 3.3). Tau proteins
are normally situated in the outer layers of the neuron, where
they promote and stabilize the assembly of structural fibers
called microtubules. In doing this, they help to organize the
structure inside the cell and provide pathways for molecules
to travel along when moving within the cell. The tau proteins
found in neurofibrillary tangles are "hyperphosphorylated,"
which means that they have several phosphorous and oxygen molecules tacked on. Hyperphosphorylation reduces
the proteins' stabilizing effect in such a way that they fold
onto themselves to become paired helical filaments, allowing the microtubules to collapse. This results in a flame-
shaped mass of abnormally twisted fibers within the neuron
(hence the name "neurofibrillary tangle"). They tend to form
within larger neurons, rarely affecting small or medium-
sized neurons.

As with plaques, the presence of apoE protein appears
to play a role in neurofibrillary tangle formation, and, again,

apoE4 is the culprit. Tau proteins are able to bind to the apoE2 and apoE3 forms of apoE, but they cannot bind to apoE4. Researchers hypothesize that the binding of apoE2 or apoE3 to tau protects tau from being hyperphosphorylated by physically obstructing the areas where phosphorous and oxygen groups might otherwise bind. This keeps neurofibrillary tangle formation in check. Because tau cannot bind to apoE4, people who produce the apoE4 form of apoE protein are less protected from formation of neurofibrillary tangles than people who produce the other two forms.

One theory about the cause of Alzheimer's disease that at this time appears unrelated to the commonly seen plaques and tangles involves the metal magnesium. Magnesium is normally present in the body and has protective properties when nerve cells are injured. If there is a decrease in magnesium, some of this protective effect is lost, making nerve cells more vulnerable to death in the event of nervous system damage. Magnesium is also intimately associated with the activity of calcium in cells, and levels of magnesium need to stay relatively constant if calcium is to function properly. Because many of the biochemical processes involving magnesium play a role in nerve cell degeneration, some investigators speculate that low magnesium levels could contribute to the neural degeneration seen in dementia. A recent study showed that patients with severe Alzheimer's disease had lower levels of magnesium in their blood than control subjects. While dietary problems and mechanisms related to magnesium storage within the body make interpretation of this finding somewhat complicated, there may be some value in determining the role played by magnesium in Alzheimer's disease.

PUTTING IT ALL TOGETHER

As we have seen, Alzheimer's disease can arise from defects in one of several different genes, from the presence of the

APO E4 gene, or from other as yet undetermined causes. Despite the differences in origin, however, the course of Alzheimer's disease appears to be basically the same across the board, at least at the tissue level. Compared to healthy people of the same age, people with Alzheimer's disease show significantly higher concentrations of plaques and tangles and significantly greater neuron and synapse loss. It would make sense for one or more of these factors to lead to the symptoms of dementia that characterize Alzheimer's disease. For a long time amyloid was thought to be the central factor leading to dementia. But the presence of plaques even in nondemented elderly people called this theory into question, as does the observation that people found to have extremely high numbers of plaques do not always have particularly severe dementia, and some people with severe dementia do not have all that many plaques. Furthermore, although beta amyloid has been shown to have toxic and inhibitory effects on the growth of dendrites and axons when tested in the laboratory on brain tissue, it does not appear to be partic- ularly toxic when it is injected into animal brains by itself. Neurofibrillary tangles do correlate strongly with memory loss on several neuropsychological tests, though not with dementia severity in general. Tangles cannot be the main cause of dementia, though, since dementia is often seen in the complete absence of tangles. Neuron and synapse loss, then, as we have said, are probably the immediate causes of dementia in Alzheimer's disease. In fact, the more synapses lost, the more severe the dementia is. Synapses are probably lost due to neuronal injury, with some contributions from the deposition of amyloid.

Several factors complicate efforts to determine the se- quence of events in Alzheimer's disease. Obviously, most features of the disease cannot be detected until brain tissue is examined at autopsy. Unless an Alzheimer's patient dies of a second unrelated disorder, such as cancer, it is likely that an autopsy will not be performed until all of the lesions that characterize the disease are present. Thus no light will be shed on the question of when the lesions may have developed in relation to one another. It would be useful to try to develop a timeline for the development of Alzheimer's disease lesions based on autopsies done on Alzheimer's patients who die in the early stages of disease. Unfortunately, although doctors encourage autopsy after the death of someone with Alzheimer's in order to confirm the diagnosis, and indeed autopsies are more common for Alzheimer's disease patients than for patients who have died of other diseases, many families ask that the procedure not be done.

Another major complication is that nondemented elderly people also seem to have many of the same lesions in their brains as people with Alzheimer's disease. When the brains of young people with Alzheimer's disease and healthy people of the same age are compared, the distinctions are clear: Alzheimer's patients have neuritic plaques and neurofibrillary tangles, while the others do not. The distinctions, however, are blurred in older people. Alzheimer lesions can be found in many nondemented elderly people. If diffuse plaques of beta amyloid are counted, then approximately half of all older people have at least a few. Those who have them are also likely to have at least some neurofibrillary tangles. The neurofibrillary tangles in cognitively normal elderly people show the same structural pattern as those in people with Alzheimer's disease and appear in the same regions of the brain, but they occur in much smaller quantities than in even mild Alzheimer's disease. Some people have proposed that the presence of both diffuse plaques and neurofibrillary tangles represents an early developmental stage of Alzheimer's disease, and that the appearance of the more damaging neuritic plaques would precipitate dementia symptoms, but this has not been established. Though it is difficult to say whether the presence of Alzheimer-type lesions constitutes an early, presymptomatic form of Alzheimer's disease or simply normal aging, it is clear that at least some cognitively intact elderly people have them. This suggests that there are other factors determining whether the symptoms of dementia arise.

One idea is that some people have so many extra neurons and synapses that when they lose even a lot, they can still function normally. Though some of them may be developing plaques and tangles, the extra "cognitive reserve" helps them to compensate for their losses, preventing or delaying the onset of dementia. This could explain results from several studies suggesting that education has a protective effect against developing Alzheimer's disease. A population survey of dementia carried out in Shanghai in 1987 showed that in subjects older than age 75, there was a striking increase in the prevalence of dementia in those with no or low education compared to those with middle school educations. Several surveys conducted since then have revealed similar results in Bordeaux, France; Appignano, Italy; Stockholm, Sweden; Ashkelon, Israel; and Finland. Experts postulate that education could increase this cognitive reserve by increasing the number and/or density of synapses in certain areas of the brain, which would then permit more time to elapse between beginning of neural degeneration and outward symptoms of dementia.

With this idea in mind, researchers at the University of Kentucky studied a group of about a hundred nuns who had entered a Milwaukee convent between 1931 and 1939. The results of the study were made public in 1996. The sisters' cognitive ability as young adults was measured through analysis of autobiographies they had written before taking their religious vows, and their cognitive ability as older adults was assessed with neuropsychological tests. The brains of those nuns who died during the study were autopsied and examined for signs of Alzheimer's disease.

The investigators expected that those sisters who had low linguistic ability in early life would have low cognitive reserve and therefore be more vulnerable to Alzheimer's disease as adults. Those with high linguistic ability in early life—

a potential indicator of brain reserve—were expected to be better protected from expressing the symptoms of Alzheimer's disease, even if they had abundant neurofibrillary tangles and plaques. Ninety percent of the nuns with Alzheimer's disease confirmed at autopsy had low linguistic ability in early life, compared with only 13 percent of those without evidence of the disease. The study revealed that poor written linguistic performance in early life is a potent indicator of risk for cognitive problems, Alzheimer's disease, and brain lesions in later life. While the association between low linguistic ability and Alzheimer's disease was expected, the investigators were surprised to find so few sisters—just one, in fact—who had high linguistic ability as a young adult but nevertheless showed characteristics of Alzheimer's disease at autopsy. The cognitive reserve idea would predict that sisters with high cognitive ability in early life would still show neuropathologic lesions, even if they did not show cognitive decline (as was the case with the one sister who fit this description). Thus the researchers concluded that low linguistic ability in young adulthood may be an early symptom of subtle changes in the brain that ultimately lead to Alzheimer's disease. This could mean that the Alzheimer's disease process begins much earlier in life than previously thought, though further study will be necessary to clarify the relationship between linguistic ability in early life and disease in old age.

4. Caring for Someone with Alzheimer's Disease

Everything that an Alzheimer's disease patient has ever learned eventually fades from memory. People with the disease gradually forget how to speak, how to act, how to dress, even how to eat. As patients' judgment and ability to care for themselves deteriorate, family, friends, and medical professionals must take responsibility. Caregivers should aim to fill the final years of the lives of Alzheimer's patients with peace, pleasure, and dignity. Though people with Alzheimer's may not express appreciation for the efforts of caregivers, there is little doubt that quality of life is vastly improved for those patients fortunate enough to have people around them who can help develop a coherent plan for their financial, social, and medical welfare. In the early stages this means helping determine who will manage the patients' financial and legal affairs when they are no longer able to, ensuring adequate funding for medical costs that are bound to arise, and discussing what kind of medical care patients would like to have. Later on, when patients are less able to understand what is going on around them, good caregiving involves developing a comfortable routine including meaningful and pleasant activities.

CAREGIVING AT HOME

Over half of all people with dementia live in the community. For the first several years after diagnosis, patients can live at home and take reasonably good care of themselves, only gradually needing more assistance. Home care is the only feasible option for most families, because nursing home care is generally too expensive for long periods of time, and people with Alzheimer's disease are likely to live for several years, even after becoming almost totally dependent upon a 24-hour caregiver. Home care is a great challenge, however, and caregivers need much practical and emotional assistance from family and friends, as well as financial resources to support themselves and the patients they care for.

Families considering home care for a loved one with Alzheimer's disease should consider the costs of a caregiver giving up a job or reducing work hours to make time for home care versus the person continuing to work and using a day care program, paid companion, or visiting nurse. Some insurance policies might cover the costs of nurses' aides or other daytime care personnel; this should be investigated. Whatever the decision, families should realize that patients' needs will change as the disease progresses, and different arrangements will probably be necessary later on. Costs of future care should be considered as arrangements are made for present care.

Careful planning can make home care of people with Alzheimer's disease successful. While at first patients may require only supervision, later on they will need assistance with almost every activity of the day, and eventually will become totally dependent on caregivers. We will begin our discussion of home care with a review of communication problems and solutions that may help to improve caregiver-patient interactions in any caring situation, and then move on to more specific suggestions for managing the home care of someone with Alzheimer's disease.

Communication

Successful caring depends on good communication. None of the functions that caregivers help their patients to perform can be done easily without communication. The loss of the ability to understand others and to be understood is devastating for patients and can make management of the disease frustrating and difficult for both patients and caregivers. The quality of life for people with Alzheimer's disease can be vastly improved by prolonging effective communication—both verbal and nonverbal—between these two parties. Effective techniques can build upon patients' remaining strengths and abilities, promoting a sense of security and self-esteem. Overall, these techniques can be summarized as simplifying what is said, reducing the necessity for patients to use their memory, and helping patients maintain their dignity.

Communication in the early stages— When people are in the mild-to-moderate stages of dementia, a useful strategy is to control conversational situations. Increase the chance of successful conversational interaction by keeping social situations and exchanges as simple as possible. For example, people with Alzheimer's disease do better in one-on-one conversations than in groups. Try to sit face-to-face with them, address them by name, and establish eye contact, all of which give patients something to focus on. Turn off the TV or radio, and minimize any other noise that could be distracting. Speak slowly and distinctly to compensate for patients' reduced ability to process information. Use a low-pitched voice to convey a sense of calm and to make it easier for hearing-impaired people to understand. Pay attention to your tone of voice; try to sound pleasant and accepting. Patients can process the emotional characteristics of speech even when they can no longer understand the semantic content, and thus caregivers should avoid a demeaning tone or baby-talk type of speech pattern. People with Alzheimer's disease tend to respond to the tone and mood of social interactions more than to actual words anyway, so it is helpful to maintain a reassuring, easy-going posture and countenance. Do not talk about patients as if they are not there; it is impossible to know how much they understand. Also, learn the limits of your particular patient's attention span. Restlessness or withdrawal may be signs that it is time for a break.

Conversation should be simplified as much as possible. Short, direct, literal sentences are best. Sentences that follow the format "subject-verb-object" are the least demanding on patients' memories. For example, it is easier for patients to understand "Martin hit the ball" than "The ball was hit by Martin." The more important part of a sentence should come first ("I *saw a play* when I was in New York" instead of "When I was in New York, I *saw a play*"). Whenever possible, compound sentences should be broken up into individual ones ("I bought milk. I went to the cleaners" instead of "I bought milk and went to the cleaners"). Use common words as much as possible and avoid using pronouns, because they require patients to remember the preceding noun. Instead, repeat the proper noun (e.g., say "Warren plays football. Warren is the quarterback," *not* "Warren plays football and he's the quarterback"). Break down complex thoughts into simple phrases, and give instructions in stages, one step at a time. Whenever possible, demonstrate actions you want the patient to take. Avoid using any indirect statements, such as "Is anybody else warm?" when "Please open the window" is what is actually meant. Patients take most statements literally, so idioms such as "give a hand," "hop into bed," or "hit the hay" should be avoided, as should teasing and sarcasm.

In conversations, focus on the here and now. Eliminate dependence on memory by talking about things that are present. Whenever possible, allow patients to see and/or touch objects being discussed in addition to hearing about them. Pictures, written cues, miming, and gestures can be used to increase understanding. Try introducing new topics with informative introductory statements, such as "I'm going to tell you about Warren's football game." Begin with general statements, moving later to more specific kinds of information. Be encouraging when patients use roundabout ways of expressing themselves—calling a desk "the table with drawers" or referring to dinner as "eating time." In the first reported case of Alzheimer's disease, the patient called a cup a "milk-pourer."

Alzheimer called this semantical pattern "perplexing," but researchers today agree that such statements are an excellent way for patients to compensate for their lost ability to find the right word.

Ask only one question at a time and wait for responses. Avoid asking open-ended questions that give patients too many options and not enough verbal cues, such as "What do you want?" Instead try to ask specific yes or no or multiple-choice questions, such as "Do you want coffee or tea?" or "Do you want a sandwich?" If something is not understood, try saying it another way, as patients may require several explanations. For example, instead of repeating "Do you want some water?" over and over if it isn't understood, try "Would you like a glass of water?" or "Are you thirsty?" Try not to argue with patients. When they disagree, a useful strategy is to agree, then distract them, divert the conversation, and later gently try again with the original topic. Limit the number of negative "Don't do this" or "Don't do that" statements used with patients.

Be patient during pauses or digressions. If patients seem to have lost track of where they are after a lengthy pause, gently prompt them, ask a relevant directing question, or summarize what has been said in a conversational manner. When people with Alzheimer's disease have a word on the tip of their tongues, allow them time to think of it. Don't rush or interrupt them, and make every effort to avoid showing impatience or annoyance through facial expressions or body language. You may offer a guess if the inability to remember a word seems to frustrate a patient, or provide a correct word if a wrong one is used; if supplied words or corrections upset the patient, however, they should not be given in the future. Some people with Alzheimer's disease will correct themselves but do not seem to like being corrected; others seem to be glad for assistance with finding the right word.

In general, be quick with praise and encouragement to make patients feel accepted and cared for. Try to make meaning of statements that at first sound like nonsensical gibberish, using patients' gestures and facial expressions as clues. People with Alzheimer's disease will often understand touch better than words. Hold their hands or put your arms around them. Touches and massage are very effective for conveying affection. Remember to move slowly to avoid startling patients and to touch gently. Encourage smiling, hugs, and eye contact. Pay close attention to patients' voices, facial expressions, and gestures for clues to what they are feeling and might be trying to communicate. These nonverbal communication skills are important throughout the course of the disease, but become most important in the latest, most severe stages of dementia, when patients' verbal communication skills deteriorate dramatically.

Communication in the latest stages— At this point people with Alzheimer's disease become disoriented with respect to time and place. They fail to recognize family members and other loved ones and are unable to form new memories. Patients may be partially or completely withdrawn, unaware that they are being spoken to. Some patients do not talk at all. For those who do, the grammatical structure of utterances may remain intact, but sentence fragments, incessantly repeated words or phrases, and meaningless language with a limited vocabulary are common. Patients may show no comprehension or use of complex forms, and yes or no responses to questions may be unreliable. Even when dementia reaches this point, caregivers should continue conversing with patients in order to prevent their withdrawal. Face-to-face, eye-to-eye contact is especially important at this time since the patient relies even more on nonverbal cues. Because most patients use wheelchairs or sit most of the time, it is crucial that those talking to them sit down, squat, or bend over so their faces can be seen. Established routines and rituals should be maintained for as long as possible to keep patients calm.

Even if patients cannot understand what is going on, they will still need affection, which can easily be conveyed through body language. As before, greet patients by holding a hand, or gently touch a shoulder to help them focus attention on you. Continue to keep the tone of your voice calm, affectionate, and supportive, and use gestures and mime to promote understanding.

Perhaps the single most important key to managing the home care of someone with Alzheimer's disease is remembering to remain calm and reassuring. Caregivers should be matter-of-fact, consistent, and in good humor. Although patients will at times display behaviors that seem remarkably unusual for them, personalities remain essentially the same: passive and accepting patients will generally continue to be agreeable, and more independent, active patients tend to remain so. Try to help patients maintain their self-image and dignity by helping them to preserve their own personalities.

The Nitty-Gritty of Home Care

A number of household modifications can make the home safer and more comfortable for the patient and simplify caregiving. Items to remove include footstools, extension cords, throw rugs, and anything else that could cause tripping, as well as table lamps, vases, and other breakables that can be easily knocked over. Furniture should not be rearranged, so that surroundings will seem familiar for as long as possible. Excess clutter may be confusing, but favorite items, such as an afghan, family photo albums, and one or two special knickknacks can provide comfort and reassurance to people with Alzheimer's disease. Because patients have a tendency to misplace things, items of great value should be kept hidden from them.

Install safety latches on cabinets containing any poisonous liquids or substances that may appear edible to Alzheimer's patients. To prevent patients from attempting to cook while unsupervised, you can install devices (available at hardware stores) that lock the knobs of ovens and stoves in the "off" position. Even better, have a stop-clock shut-off valve installed in the gas feedline behind the stove. You can also turn an electric stove off at the circuit breaker. Smoking is another possible fire hazard, since someone with Alzheimer's disease may forget that a cigarette is lit and leave it someplace where a fire could start. Thus smokers should be closely supervised, and lighters and other smoking materials should be controlled by the caregiver.

The family car is another potential danger. Early in the disease you may be able to tactfully discuss driving with the affected person, who may voluntarily agree to stop driving. However, this is difficult for most people, since driving is such a visible symbol of freedom and individual responsibility in American society. At some point, however, it will be absolutely necessary to prevent someone with Alzheimer's disease from driving. You may need to ask for help from a family physician, who can write a "prescription" saying "Do not drive." Patients are often more willing to listen to authority figures on this issue. Even so, you should always keep tabs on the car keys, and, if necessary, learn quick and easily reversible ways to disable the car, such as removing the distributor cap.

Establishing a routine will help make patients feel comfortable. Signs describing the regular activities of each day and the times they occur can be posted on the refrigerator for easy reference. Large clocks and calendars on the wall can help to orient patients to time of day and season. Repeat names of people frequently to help patients identify them, and announce each activity or action before beginning it. Give oral instructions slowly, and put up written instructions for activities that are done on a daily basis.

Suggested daily activities— Each day should begin with orienting activities to help patients to remember who and where they are and what they will be doing that day. The caregiver might say something like, "Good morning, Michael, I'm your wife, Susan, and I'm going to be helping you today. It's Wednesday, March 22, and it's a beautiful sunny day. We will be going for a walk this morning to look at all the blooming flowers." Some caregivers like to give a daily tour of their patient's surroundings, naming each room and what is done there, pointing out prominently posted lists of activities, identifying loved ones who appear in photographs, etc. Orienting activities are often useful in the evenings as well, because, as it becomes dark, some people seem to experience more confusion and agitation in a phenomenon known as "sundowning." It's a good idea to draw the blinds at night, because people often mistake their reflection in the window for a stranger outside, and become anxious. Drawing the blinds can become part of a set of evening rituals that might include playing quiet music, sharing a warm drink, and turning on a night light. Caregivers may want to point out that darkness is the time for putting on pajamas and staying in bed with lights out.

During the day, there are many kinds of activities that can be done with people who have Alzheimer's disease. For as long as possible, people should be encouraged to continue hobbies and activities they practiced when they were well. If they liked playing a musical instrument or dancing, for example, they may continue to enjoy these activities long into the illness. If the loss of cognitive ability makes a previously enjoyed activity too difficult to carry out, so that it becomes frustrating, the activity should be discouraged or modified in such a way that patients can feel successful while doing it. For example, a simple form of embroidery with large blocks of single colors can be satisfying for someone who used to enjoy counted cross-stitch embroidery, and word searches might be suitable replacements for crossword puzzles. Alzheimer's patients may enjoy crafts, painting, simple games, and jigsaw puzzles. Children's games are often suitable activities but should be modified for adults—some people with Alzheimer's disease may feel they are being treated as children and become resentful. For example, the completion of a jigsaw puzzle may be satisfying for someone, but as the disease progresses the puzzles offered need to be simpler with fewer pieces. Unfortunately, such puzzles tend to have pictures that are designed to amuse children; instead, one that depicts a landscape or famous painting would be more appropriate for the adult who will be working it. Other simple games perceived as adult games, such as shuffleboard, can be immensely enjoyable for patients.

People with Alzheimer's disease often like to be helpful and should be encouraged to assist with household chores to the extent that they are able. Helping to make the beds, dust the house, and sweep the floor are examples of potentially enjoyable activities that can be worked into everyday routines. Furthermore, some people feel useful if they are given a task to do, such as folding a pile of newly washed towels, and will enjoy folding, unfolding, and refolding the towels repeatedly. While this kind of repetition seems like a waste of time to healthy people, if patients enjoy such activities and are not creating any disturbance, there is nothing wrong with permitting the practice.

Working some kind of exercise into each day is a good idea. Possibilities include walks through the neighborhood, stretches to music, and dancing. Gardening, an activity that many people find enjoyable, can provide a good amount of exercise.

Visitors can and should be included in any of these types of activities. In fact, it is often better to have visitors participate in enjoyable activities such as sing-alongs or exercise sessions than to simply talk. Especially later on in the disease, conversation becomes more and more difficult, which can be discomfiting for the visitor and frustrating for the patient. Children, with their happy and usually unembarrassed natures, make especially good visitors. Teenagers tend to be more embarrassed, but can overcome this if they are distracted from the illness and made to focus on the activity they are sharing with the patient. People with Alzheimer's disease also tend to enjoy pets if they did so before the disease, especially because animals provide loyal companionship without regard to their owners' cognitive abilities. Nervous or loud animals should be avoided, as they may cause confusion or agitation, and, to prevent the patient's tripping, all pets should be trained not to get underfoot. Though caring for both pet and patient may prove to be too much work for a single caregiver, pets can greatly improve the quality of life for someone with Alzheimer's disease if the necessary support is there.

In short, any activities that are reassuring and don't cause confusion are appropriate for people with Alzheimer's disease. Emphasize patients' remaining capabilities for as long as possible and reinforce their positive behaviors.

Mealtimes— Mealtimes can be overwhelming for people with Alzheimer's disease, because of all the details that need to be remembered—how to use utensils, how to chew and swallow, what to eat first—not to mention remembering that they need to eat in the first place. Caregivers should keep mealtime simple. Serve food with as few utensils as possible, and try serving only one part of a meal at a time. Caregivers may need to demonstrate how to chew or swallow on occasion. Finger foods are often helpful when utensil use is a problem. If patients forget that they have recently eaten and request more food, healthy snacks such as cheese slices or crackers can come in handy. Patients who enjoy drinking alcoholic beverages may be permitted to continue this habit, although it's best not to encourage them. Cocktails should be mixed by caregivers, since patients might misjudge the amount of alcohol they are serving themselves, and servings should be limited to one a day, preferably with a meal.

Grooming— People with Alzheimer's disease can be helped to recognize that each morning represents a new day of activity by being encouraged to maintain their former standard of personal hygiene. Patients feel good when they look good, and visitors respond better to people who look their best. Simplify the grooming routine as much as possible. Install nonskid mats and grab bars in the bathroom to allow patients to bathe themselves in private. When supervision becomes required, as it eventually will, both patients and caregivers will have to adjust to the new lack of privacy. Caregivers should be matter-of-fact instead of embarrassed, providing reassurance while supervising and, later on, while bathing the person. Alzheimer's patients may also resist bathing. To avoid this problem, make bathing a part of the regular routine; say, "It's time for your bath" instead of "You need a bath." The latter statement implies that something is wrong with the person, which may cause agitation. It is easier to make "time" the reason for the bath. Male patients should receive help shaving at least every few days.

Make sure that the grooming routine includes toothbrushing and flossing, and arrange for regular dental checkups. Cavities and other basic dental problems are twice as common in Alzheimer's patients as in healthy people of the same age, and can cause larger problems if not discovered early on. For example, a toothache may cause agitation or a refusal to eat, and a patient might be unable to communicate what the cause is. Further, the measures necessary to correct a toothache or gum problem once it has been diagnosed are even more stressful for people with Alzheimer's disease than they are for everyone else. Prevention is the watchword here.

Provide loose-fitting but stylish clothing that is easy to put on—avoid buttons or zippers wherever possible. Do not give patients too many choices of what to wear, as this might be overwhelming. Women who normally wear make-up and accessories should be encouraged to continue this practice to maintain their self-esteem and image. When it becomes necessary to dress and groom patients, describing each step and admiring the results can have a reassuring effect.

Toileting— Caregivers should learn the toilet habits of their patients. While most people with Alzheimer's disease are able to recognize that they need to use the bathroom at least until the later stages of disease, they may have difficulty locating the bathroom or using it once they are there. A sign on the bathroom door showing a picture of a toilet and the word "bathroom" can help. Also, caregivers should watch for signals such as restlessness, wandering, or tugging at clothing, so that a trip to the bathroom may be suggested just in case. Later on most patients do become incontinent, and a schedule for changing of incontinence clothing will be necessary. Accidents should be handled matter-of-factly. Praise patients when they are successful, but do not scold them when they are not.

Medications— Many older people take medications for various underlying illnesses, such as high blood pressure, diabetes, heart disease, and arthritis, that will need to be monitored carefully in someone with Alzheimer's disease. Caregivers will have to dispense the medications at the appropriate times and monitor reactions. Patients may experience sedating, intoxicating, or otherwise disturbing effects from sedatives, analgesics, tranquilizers, antidepressants, or combinations of these drugs with any other medications they are taking. It is best for Alzheimer's patients to have one physician coordinating all prescribed medications. If more than one doctor is involved, it is vital to ensure that each doctor knows about all of the patient's medications.

Behavior Problems— Due to the nature of Alzheimer's disease, problems ranging from the mildly annoying to the out-and-out dangerous will arise. Even the most experienced and knowledgeable caregivers have problems, and most people caring for Alzheimer's patients are not experienced or knowledgeable when they begin. It is important to remember that patients do not intend to be difficult, and that outbursts or other problems are the results of a disease over which they have no control. Alzheimer's disease gradually destroys all learned behaviors—including manners and sensitivity—so problems are bound to come up. Anticipating difficult behaviors helps to avoid some problems and eases to some degree the ones that do occur.

Wandering is a frequently reported behavioral problem comprising a patient's pacing around a room, following the caregiver from room to room, or simply walking off. Since they lose their memory of familiar landmarks, patients can be lost in their own front yards, so it is important not to leave them unattended outside. In situations where there are several people present in the home, make sure that one person is clearly responsible for knowing where the Alzheimer's patient is. Some families have members take turns with this responsibility. Patients should wear Medic-Alert bracelets with their addresses on them in case they do get lost somewhere, and caregivers and/or families should keep recent photos of patients on hand in case the police must be called in to help search. To prevent someone from leaving at night when caregivers are not watching, install a deadbolt lock on the main door of the house, or add a lock to the door in a place a patient might not think to look, such as near the floor.

If wandering occurs at a specific time of day, it may be reduced by the undertaking of a more strenuous activity, such as a long walk, immediately before that time. If wandering coincides with a particular event each day, such as mealtime or the arrival of a particular person, caregivers should try to make that event less stressful in case the wandering represents an effort to escape the situation. If wandering occurs at night, more exercise during the day may help the person to sleep through the night. Since wandering may also represent a search for the bathroom, caregivers should ask patients if they need to use the bathroom.

People with Alzheimer's disease may suffer from *delusions* or *hallucinations*. Delusions are incorrect beliefs that persist despite their irrationality; an example would be a female patient believing that she is pregnant. Hallucinations are sensory experiences that clearly are not real; the patient might, for instance, believe that he or she is seeing someone who is not actually there. If the person does not appear to be upset by these disturbances, allow them to persist. If the person is upset or frightened, though, acknowledge the fear and reassure him or her that you are there to make things right. Distraction is always a useful tactic. Be noncommittal if the patient wants to discuss what he or she has seen or heard. Do not acknowledge the truth or deny the reality of what the patient perceives. If hallucinations or delusions become more troubling, drug treatment is also a possibility (see chapter 5).

Alzheimer's patients may display a variety of inappropriate or annoying behaviors, including making tactless or insulting remarks or unreasonable demands or complaints, using foul language, repeating questions or actions, dressing improperly, acting childish, or performing sexually explicit acts. Most often the best way to deal with these behaviors is to distract the person with an acceptable activity, then offer praise and positive reinforcement. Scolding, arguing, or trying to teach people with Alzheimer's disease how to act properly are not effective strategies. Tactless remarks or insults may reflect patients' fears or uncertainties, and indicate that they need reassurance. If a patient complains, for example, that you are never there when she needs you, when in fact you are there 24 hours a day, instead of pointing this out you might say sympathetically, "I know you worry when you can't see me." If a patient makes unreasonable demands, try setting schedules and time limits. Timers, in fact, are a good way to bring about endings to activities. If repetitive actions are not harmful or inappropriate, they should be allowed. Repeated questions may reflect a patient's nervousness or inability to think of anything else to say. Rather than answering the question the same way every time, you might reassure patients that everything is fine and distract them with another activity. If patients try to undress, make sure that their clothes are comfortable, and that they do not need to use the bathroom. Sexually explicit actions are actually quite rare and sometimes are not really sexual in nature but rather fidgety behaviors, such as repeatedly zipping or unzipping a fly or blouse. The best strategy is to direct the person to another activity.

Some people with Alzheimer's disease enjoy hoarding small items or rummaging in boxes with such contents. A box or drawer of objects that can be fiddled with may provide for a person's need to do this without his or her disturbing items that are necessary for the running of the household.

Catastrophic reaction is a term used to describe any strenuously difficult reaction to an overwhelming situation. Anger, stubbornness, combativeness and agitation may be part of such reactions. To avoid them, don't force people with Alzheimer's disease to participate in anything. Avoid crowds, strangers, and claustrophobic conditions, as well as clutter, confusion or noise. If a particular activity seems to cause frequent catastrophic reactions, avoid that activity or redesign it to be less stressful. When these reactions do happen, stay calm. Announce your actions in advance and move slowly. Do not touch the patient in any way that would suggest restraint. Do not discuss the event either; take advantage of the patient's forgetfulness.

Caregivers need to keep expectations realistic. The people in their care will not get better, but with good caregiving Alzheimer's patients can maintain their independence and dignity for a long time. Caregivers need to be prepared for problem behaviors and to be tolerant when such behaviors arise. Flexibility is also important. The situation will change from day to day. What worked yesterday may not work today.

But with patience and understanding, caregiving can be a rewarding experience.

Maintaining a calm environment and prolonging effective communication between Alzheimer's patients and caregivers is a daunting task. The techniques discussed here can be useful, but even then there will be times when patients and caregivers are frustrated. Caregivers may feel guilty when they communicate poorly, show impatience, or fail to remain calm. It is important to remember that very few people (if any) can maintain a perfect demeanor when they care for someone around the clock. There will be days when caregiving seems impossible. The techniques presented here may help to ease the difficulties somewhat, enabling people with Alzheimer's disease to use whatever cognitive skills they retain for as long as possible.

RESPITE AND NURSING HOME CARE

Caregivers are only human and need to take breaks from what is a very taxing and stressful job. There are several avenues that enable caregivers to have some time off while ensuring adequate care for their charges. In families where the primary caregiver is a family member, the most obvious solution is often for another family member to provide care once or twice a week, even if only for a few hours. Regularly scheduled absences of the primary caregiver can be worked into the patient's weekly routine. To reassure someone with Alzheimer's that the caregiver will come back, it is often helpful to leave behind a note telling when to expect his or her return. Another solution that allows the primary caregiver regular resting periods is to hire visiting health care professionals one or two days a week. Adult day care is a third alternative that permits caregivers a day or two off a week. The number of adult (often called "senior") day care centers specializing in dementing illnesses is rapidly increasing; these are a boon to patients and their families. Though programs vary widely, most centers provide a wide range of meaningful activities aimed at people with different levels of impairment, while also caring for their physical needs.

At some point, the primary caregiver will probably want (and need!) to take an extended vacation. Trusted family members or friends may be willing to provide care for a week or two, but for this option to be successful, it is important that the substitute caregiver be aware of and prepared for the demands of the job. Having a health care professional live in may be preferable; a trained person is more likely to understand the demands and be familiar with the kinds of problems that may arise. If the substitute has spent some time helping with care in the past, however, it can be reassuring for a person to receive care from someone the patient already knows, such as a family member, who is familiar with the basic routine.

Some hospitals and nursing facilities will admit patients for short-term stays so that caregivers can take extended vacations. While such stays may be somewhat disorienting to people with Alzheimer's disease, it is generally agreed that the benefits for the primary caregiver—improved health and outlook—may contribute to the quality of overall caregiving and ultimately outweigh the drawbacks of such a plan.

Eventually, the question of long-term nursing home placement will come up. If a spouse or family member is the primary caregiver, there will come a point when the patient's behavior begins to be too difficult to handle. Caregivers start to question whether or not they are capable of continuing this job alone. Caring for loved ones who are no longer the people they used to be can be quite painful. As much as caregivers love the people they care for, the changes that must be endured are extremely stressful. Making matters worse is a dramatic deterioration in the quality of caregivers' social lives. In situations where medical problems are acute, family and friends are likely to rally around ill patients and their immediate families, whereas when the illness is chronic and progressive, as in Alzheimer's disease, people are frequently too uncomfortable about the situation to come around often. As a result, caregivers may feel abandoned by people who were once close friends. Their activities become more and more constrained to the point where they can hardly make trips to the market, the barber, or even the bathroom. Patients can't converse anymore, and the monotony of doing the same things day after day often becomes difficult to bear. Caregivers become angrier with patients and about their own situation. Sometimes it is nearly impossible for a person to avoid snapping at a difficult patient, and this may cause guilt, but neither is it healthy to hold such feelings inside.

Although many caregivers feel guilty about putting loved ones in a nursing home, and angry that such a choice even needs to be made, it is often the only option left. Most caregivers report that any resentment they felt toward the person they cared for dissipates when they relinquish the responsibility of round-the-clock care; thus caregivers are able to have better relationships with their loved ones. In a good nursing home, the physical needs of Alzheimer's disease patients are provided for in a cheerful, confident manner without sorrow or anger. This kind of caregiving becomes progressively more and more difficult for a nonprofessional—particularly a family member—to carry out.

On average, Alzheimer's patients are placed in nursing homes or similar facilities two years after diagnosis, and remain there for just under four years. It is wise to begin research of nearby nursing facilities early in the course of the disease, as there are often waiting lists for the few available beds. There are many questions to consider in the search for an appropriate home. Type of facility is one consideration. Some nursing facilities take Alzheimer's or dementia patients exclusively, whereas others have special Alzheimer's disease programs or care units within a more diverse population of residents. The severity of disease in your particular patient will in part determine which type of facility is best for you. Some people with Alzheimer's disease require assistance with every activity of the day—from getting out of bed to bathing to eating to walking around—while others are more independent. Some nursing facilities are better equipped than others to care for more severely demented people. It will be necessary to determine which facilities are up to providing the level of care appropriate for your patient.

Cost and location are two other extremely important considerations. How much does each facility cost, and how will it be possible to meet these costs? How many spaces are available at each home, and how long does the typical person have to wait before being admitted? Is the facility near enough to permit frequent visits by family members or by the patient's physician if the family decides to retain the same one?

After some of these basic questions have been answered and a list has been made, families should visit each of the facilities they are considering. At the facility, they should interview an administrator, such as the head of nursing or of social work, who will be able to provide a tour and answer any questions. Some families are impressed by fancy, well-decorated facilities and put off by more simple, functional surroundings. Keep in mind that Alzheimer's patients probably won't know the difference, and that care and staff quality are far more important. As long as the building is reasonably clean, with well-lit, uncluttered walkways and comfortable homey rooms, furniture and decor should not be a major concern.

Time the visit for late morning; at this time of day, residents should be out of bed, dressed and groomed. Ask to watch residents eating lunch, and note how much assistance and individual attention is given to those who need it. Observe staff interactions with residents in general to ensure that patients are treated respectfully and as adults who happen to be ill rather than as children or people not worth talking to.

Also compare the staff-to-resident ratio, and find out whether or not the number of staff members decreases at night or on holidays.

Find out what kind of recreation programs the facility offers. Clocks, calendars, and schedules of activities should be visible to orient residents as to where they are and what they are doing, and staff should wear name tags. Recreation programs might include musical activities, viewing of suitable television programs or videos, outdoor walks, exercise classes, arts and crafts, and even activities that seem like chores but that may make residents feel useful, such as helping to make beds or fold linens. Other issues to consider include emergency medical arrangements, procedures for handling behavioral problems such as wandering, policy on sedative or restraint use, and visiting hours for family, physicians, and clergy.

It is often wise to speak with the staff member who is responsible for dealing with financial issues and can show you the contract that would be signed in the event you decided to bring your loved one to the facility. Find out what services are covered in the basic fee, what services cost extra, and how often payment is expected.

As the list is narrowed down, you may wish to pay second visits to some of the better facilities. You should not feel embarrassed or fussy to be doing this; after all, you want to choose the home that will best serve the needs of someone you care about. Being certain that a particular facility is right for your patient will prevent your having to further disrupt your loved one's life by moving him or her to another facility later.

LEGAL AND FINANCIAL MATTERS

It is important to consult a lawyer when someone has been diagnosed with Alzheimer's disease. A variety of issues will need to be worked out to assure legal protection for patients and their assets. Many important concerns will need to be discussed by patients and their families, with decisions being made as early as possible, because most legal procedures are simpler if they are conducted while patients are still competent. Keep in mind that a diagnosis of Alzheimer's disease does not mean that people are unable to think for themselves; most people in the early stages of Alzheimer's disease are able to make important decisions even if they have difficulty managing some of their day-to-day affairs, and they should be encouraged to maintain as much control over their life and affairs as possible.

Families may begin their search for good legal advice with an attorney they have worked with before, who may refer them to someone with more expertise in the area if necessary. The local chapter of the Alzheimer's Disease and Related Disorders Association (ADRDA) may be able to suggest local lawyers with expertise in the areas that are important for Alzheimer's disease patients, as might local or state bar associations, legal aid societies, and of course, family and friends. Because laws vary from state to state, and because everyone's financial and legal situation is different, it is extremely important for families to locate this kind of legal advice as early as possible.

Once a consultation has been set up, it is useful to bring as many pertinent legal and financial documents as possible. This includes all wills and trusts, recent tax returns, health and life insurance policies, information on pension plans, IRAs, and annuity plans, deeds, mortgages, bank and credit union account information, descriptions of any potential employee benefit plans, and information on any financial investments. It can also be helpful to bring a list of organiza-tions that the Alzheimer's disease patient has been affiliated with, such as church groups, service organizations, labor unions, and military organizations, because some of these groups might assist with costs or provide services. A good legal consultant may be able to get information on some of these programs.

Managing Financial Concerns

Power of attorney— Perhaps the most useful action someone with Alzheimer's disease can take is to assign power of attorney to a spouse, child, or other close relative or trusted friend. Power of attorney allows one person (called the *principal*) to give another person (the *agent* or *attorney in fact*) the power to make decisions regarding his or her health or estate. Power of attorney can be broad, allowing the agent to control almost all of the principal's affairs, or it can be limited to certain activities only. In a few states, power of attorney becomes null and void when the principal becomes incompetent, but most states have *durable power of attorney*, which lasts until the principal has died. Durable power of attorney may become effective immediately, or not until the principal loses capacity, depending on what the document itself specifies. A more specific type of durable power of attorney, the *durable power of attorney for health care*, permits the agent to make decisions regarding only the health care of the principal.

Living trust— Also called the *inter vivos*, a living trust permits an individual (the *grantor* or *settlor*) to appoint a trustee to manage assets that have been placed in a trust according to the terms of the trust. Often the grantor serves as the trustee until he or she is no longer able, and then a previously appointed successor takes over. One advantage of living trusts is that their use avoids the necessity for an estate to go through probate, a costly and time-consuming legal process that determines how an estate will be distributed. There are other kinds of trusts that may be helpful in certain situations; a *supplemental needs trust*, for example, holds and permits use of money that normally might disqualify someone from receiving Medicaid or other forms of public assistance.

Conservatorship of property— If no durable power of attorney has been assigned, then when someone with Alzheimer's disease is no longer able to manage his or her assets, the court may appoint someone to act as *conservator*. Generally this is done after family members or other interested parties petition the court to do so. The management of assets is then monitored by the court. Sometimes this process presents difficulties; thus, whenever possible durable power of attorney should be used to maximize flexibility for families of people with Alzheimer's disease.

Property transfer— Many people with Alzheimer's disease transfer the title of any properties they own to family members or friends who can better manage the property. Such transfers need to be carefully considered for their impact on taxes and public assistance benefits. Bank accounts should also be modified to permit other people (family members and/or agent with power of attorney) to draw funds when patients are no longer competent to do so.

Tax returns— Tax returns can be done by power of attorney if specified by the power of attorney document. This is usually unnecessary for married patients, who can simply file jointly with a spouse.

Will— Fairly early on after diagnosis of Alzheimer's disease, a patient's will should be located and modified, if necessary, or drawn up if that has not been done. Unlike a trust, a will does not necessarily avoid probate, so it is wise to have both trusts and a will.

Medical costs— Medical costs on top of regular costs of living can be enormous in the later stages of Alzheimer's disease. Families should investigate the patient's health insurance policies and employment benefits to determine what avenues of funding may be available. Some insurance policies and pension plans will pay disability benefits to people with Alzheimer's disease. Many plans, however, do not adequately cover long-term care and exclude in-home care reimbursement and coverage for preexisting conditions. There are several government sources that can be helpful, both in providing supplemental income, which is important if the patient does not have any kind of retirement benefits and/or the spouse must quit working to care for the patient, and in providing help with direct medical costs.

Social Security Disability provides aid to wage earners under the age of 65 who cannot work because they are disabled. Simply having Alzheimer's disease does not make someone disabled; applicants must prove that they cannot work, which depends in large part on the stage of the disease. Therefore, many first-time applicants to the program are denied assistance, but most people can successfully appeal the decision, especially as the disease worsens. Payments are based on past salaries. Another source of income is Supplemental Security Income (SSI), which guarantees a minimum monthly income to people who are over the age of 65, disabled, or blind and with limited income. In this program, payments for those who are over 65 may be greater than for those who claim disability, so Alzheimer's disease patients over 65 should base their claim on their age and not on their disability. It is possible to qualify for SSI even with some financial assets, including a home and modest income. People who qualify for SSI also qualify for Medicaid automatically in most states (see below). General Public Assistance is a third, albeit extremely limited, source of income that may help people who do not qualify for other forms of assistance or who are waiting for other forms to begin.

Direct medical costs can be met with assistance from Medicare and Medicaid programs. Medicare is a federal health insurance program for all Americans over the age of 65 who are receiving Social Security retirement benefits. People under the age of 65 who have received Social Security Disability benefits for over a year also qualify. Medicare covers inpatient hospital care and some skilled nursing care, but does not cover long-term residential care. Also, some doctors may not accept Medicare rates for services, so families should inquire about a doctor's policies regarding Medicare before taking people with Alzheimer's disease in for treatment. Medicaid is a federal aid program administered by individual states, so eligibility and benefits vary widely. Medicaid sometimes covers the cost of long-term residential care, but often not until the patient's personal assets have run out. (Generally a home is not considered a personal asset in determining eligibility.) Alternative avenues should therefore be used whenever possible to avoid impoverishing the family members who survive someone with Alzheimer's disease. It is nice to know, however, that if it becomes necessary, Medicaid guarantees a minimum monthly payment to the spouse of an Alzheimer's disease patient. Again, some facilities will not accept Medicaid patients, a factor that should be considered by whoever is selecting an appropriate program (see discussion below).

Other organizations that may offer monetary assistance to members and sometimes nonmembers include labor unions, church groups, and fraternal organizations. Programs run by local agencies, such as Meals on Wheels, home repair programs, and free transportation programs, may also defray costs to individual families.

Managing Health Care Decisions

Living will and power of attorney— A living will is a document that describes an individual's wishes regarding artificial lifesaving measures. Basically, it provides some basis for physicians to decide how to care for patients who can no longer be involved in decision making. As mentioned earlier, power of attorney is another way to approach this issue, with individuals designating agents to make health-care decisions in their stead. Patients should discuss their wishes with their families and the agents selected to have power of attorney so that appropriate decisions can be made.

Guardianship or conservatorship of person— Like the conservatorship of property, this is a court proceeding that appoints legal guardians for patients when they become unable to care for themselves. It is usually only necessary for people who have no family to care for them.

COPING

Coping with Alzheimer's disease is not easy. Caregiving is so universally recognized as being difficult that caregivers are sometimes referred to as "second victims" of Alzheimer's disease. It's easy for caregivers to feel lonely and isolated; as the people being cared for deteriorate, the demands of caregiving increase, and the changes in lifestyle often result in fewer social contacts. Furthermore, research shows that both the emotional and the physical health of caregivers tend to be negatively affected by the stresses of caring for someone full-time. Caregivers report higher rates of depression and dissatisfaction with life in general than do average people with similar backgrounds. Several studies have shown that these stresses can even lead to impaired immune functioning, so that caregivers become more vulnerable to colds and other, mostly minor, illnesses that only add to the strain. While this research does not mean that caregivers will invariably become ill or suffer from major depression, it is clear that caregiving is an immense burden for anyone to bear. Caregivers need to take measures to avoid becoming secondary victims of Alzheimer's disease.

A number of programs in the community can help. Caregivers can join family support groups, many of which are sponsored by the Alzheimer's Disease and Related Disorders

Association. This is a nonprofit organization dedicated to supporting Alzheimer's research, developing public education programs, and providing assistance and education to Alzheimer's patients and their families, caregivers, and health care providers. Support groups led by professionals or by peers consist of caregivers, family members and friends of people with Alzheimer's disease. They meet once or twice a month at hospitals, churches, libraries, nursing homes, senior centers, or private homes and allow people with similar experiences to interact and support each other. Some groups meet regularly and focus on sharing experiences and brainstorming ideas for solving problems; other groups may be educational in nature and only last for several weeks. Educational courses are often run by professionals and vary considerably in their goals. Some educate caregivers about dementia and the process of caring, inform caregivers about community resources and available services, and provide additional information regarding various items of interest, including legal concerns, nutrition, and behavior management. Others teach specific psychologic and behavioral skills to caregivers to enhance coping and problem-solving skills. Still others may be more focused on teaching techniques to use with patients, or for caregivers themselves, in such areas as stress release, relaxation, and self-esteem improvement, all of which can greatly ease the burden of caregiving. Some cities even have specialized support groups for various groups of affected people, such as adolescents, adult children caring for parents, spouses, and widows or widowers.

The great advantage of attending a support group is that caregivers realize they are not alone. Support groups can provide new circles of friends, people who understand what caregivers and family members are going through. At meetings caregivers can feel free to express their true feelings about what they are going through in an open, caring environment. They can vent frustrations and disappointments, as well as share their successes. Furthermore, people in the support group can learn from one another, discussing such matters as behavioral management, details on nearby day care programs, or listings of area doctors who are familiar with dementia.

Aside from making use of whatever supportive resources are available locally, perhaps the most important coping technique is developing a positive attitude about the caregiving situation. Caregivers need to remember that they cannot cure the person they care for, and that there will be problems that are out of their control. They should focus on changing what can be changed, and be realistic about what they are capable of doing. They should arrange to take time out for a special evening or shopping trip to reward themselves for a job well done. Despite all of the difficulties inherent in caring for someone with Alzheimer's disease, there is a positive side. Nearly three-fourths of caregivers report that caregiving makes them feel useful, and that they are glad for the opportunity to spend time with a loved one, whose life will be made meaningful and pleasant for as long as possible. Caregiving often improves the relationship between caregiver and care recipient, and can contribute to increased self-esteem in the caregiver.

5. Treatments for Alzheimer's Disease

Trying to find treatments for Alzheimer's disease is a daunting challenge. Because the underlying causes of the disease are still so poorly understood, we have not yet developed a cure nor even treatments that reliably slow the progression of the disease. Even so, some therapies can assist in the management of many disease symptoms, and a number of potential treatments are currently being investigated. In this chapter we will review the available therapies.

PSYCHIATRIC AND BEHAVIORAL TREATMENTS

Although memory loss is what people think of first when they think of Alzheimer's disease, dramatic behavioral changes are also universal. Many of the difficult behaviors shown by people with Alzheimer's disease, and constructive ideas for dealing with them, have been discussed in the previous chapter on caregiving. Psychosocial interventions—simple things like redirecting the patient's attention during a hallucination—are often sufficient to avert serious problems. Some symptoms may stem from underlying depression or other psychoses, and many can be alleviated with drug therapy. Diagnosing these problems, however, is not as straightforward in people with Alzheimer's disease as it is in other people. We will review some of the different depressive syndromes and psychoses seen in those with Alzheimer's disease and offer recommendations for treatment. While there are many therapies available for these illnesses, special care must be taken to select drugs that are appropriate for Alzheimer's patients. The regimen should be tailored to the psychiatric symptoms of each individual, and medications that could have a negative impact on the course of Alzheimer's should be avoided. For example, medications that deplete stores of the neurotransmitter acetylcholine should be avoided in people with Alzheimer's, as they may make cognitive problems worse. Furthermore, the special problems posed by treatment of elderly people in general must be taken into consideration. In particular, many elderly people require medication for other chronic medical conditions such as hypertension or arthritis. Because negative side effects are more likely to occur if patients are taking more than one kind of drug, doctors must be careful to prescribe drugs that are less likely to interact and cause problems. The therapeutic regimen should be regularly assessed for effectiveness and lack of negative side effects and adjusted when necessary. Of course, drug therapy should be combined with social and/or behavioral programs.

Depression

Depression occurs in one-third to one-half of all people with Alzheimer's disease. While depression in younger people is frequently thought of as a condition in which someone is sad or "blue," depression in older people can occur without this particular symptom. Other good clues that someone might be depressed include a general loss of interest or ability to feel pleasure, changes in appetite and sleep, loss of energy, feelings of worthlessness or guilt, and decreased concentration. A wide range of these symptoms may occur in Alzheimer's disease patients; some can be treated with drugs, others can be treated more simply.

For example, in early stage Alzheimer's disease, most patients go through a grieving process during which they become sad because they are aware of their declining cognitive abilities. Such sadness is normal and does not require drug

treatment. However, sadness accompanied by a serious loss
of self-esteem, slowing of reaction time, or talk of suicide
is probably not just part of grieving, or simply "the blues,"
but is a sign of a major depressive episode. Mild depressive
syndromes characterized by sad mood, motor activity slowing,
hopeless or helpless feelings, crying, and/or anxiety are also
common in Alzheimer's disease. When these symptoms are
mild, they do not usually need to be treated. Though they
may be distressing to the patient, they tend to go away as
mental function deteriorates. It is also worth noting that
in Alzheimer's populations, unlike in healthy populations,
poor sleep and reduced appetite are not necessarily reliable
indicators of depression, because the disease itself may cause
these symptoms without the presence of underlying depression. It is also important to remember that depression in
Alzheimer's disease patients may not involve crying or a sad
mood; symptoms may be limited to a slowing of reaction
time or preoccupation with bodily health, perhaps as a way
of denying the loss of mental health.

Major depression occurs in about 10 percent of people with
Alzheimer's disease and is characterized by a sudden deterioration in appetite, sleep, energy, and interest. These people
may frequently talk about dying. This type of depression
may be successfully treated with antidepressant medication
(see appendix B). Often prescribed are some of the more
recently developed antidepressants, including fluoxetine
(Prozac®), sertraline (Zoloft®), paroxetine (Paxil®), venlafax-
ine (Effexor®), and bupropion (Wellbutrin®). These drugs
generally have few side effects, although headaches, nausea,
insomnia, nervousness and loss of appetite may occur with
fluoxetine, sertraline or paroxetine. Tricyclic antidepressants,
an older class of antidepressants, are also considered safe for
use in Alzheimer's disease but must be used with caution
as they may cause lightheadedness, dizziness, nausea, and
sedation. Drugs in this class such as nortriptyline (Aventyl®
or Pamelor®) and desipramine (Norpramin® or Pertofrane®)

may be safer and have fewer side effects than amitriptyline (Elaril®) or imipramine (Tofraril®), although the latter can be very useful occasionally in low dosage.

Depressive symptoms may also come from coexisting illnesses such as hypothyroidism or from medications such as digitalis and a variety of drugs given for high blood pressure. Depression caused by illness or medication is known as secondary depression. It is best managed by diagnosing and treating the underlying cause, such as by reducing or stopping treatment with an offending medication. If depression persists despite these measures, *then* therapy with antidepressant can be tried.

Anxiety and agitation

People with Alzheimer's disease may at times appear anxious and will very likely at one time or another become agitated. Agitation comprises physical restlessness—such as pacing or continual hand-wringing—as well as more difficult behaviors including extreme excitation, uncooperativeness, or argumentativeness. *Primary agitation* is related to Alzheimer's disease directly, whereas *secondary agitation* stems from depression or other psychiatric disorders that are more readily treated. Often agitation can be managed simply by speaking calmly to patients, providing reassurances that they are all right. When symptoms persist or seem to be causing undue stress, agitation may be treated with drugs designed to treat anxiety (e.g., lorazepam [Ativan®] or buspirone [Buspar®]), or, in more severe cases, low doses of drugs designed to treat psychotic illnesses (see appendix B). Many caregivers do not like the idea of using tranquilizing drugs on their patients, but short-term use is not harmful and can improve quality of life. Even so, such treatment is not always beneficial and should only be considered after behavioral interventions have been unsuccessful.

Psychotic symptoms

Many people with Alzheimer's disease experience psychotic symptoms with the advancing severity of their illness. The most common of these symptoms in Alzheimer's disease include paranoid delusions (e.g., patients believe that someone is stealing from them or plotting against them), misidentification syndromes (e.g., patients fail to recognize familiar people or things, believe people on TV are actually present, confuse strangers with family members), and hallucinatory experiences (i.e., patients see or hear things that are not actually there). Hallucinations are rarely as bizarre as they might be in psychoses such as schizophrenia; more often they relate to earlier times in the person's life. For example, a patient may start talking about business with a former coworker when no one is actually present. Approximately 30 percent of people with Alzheimer's disease exhibit some kind of paranoia in the early stages of disease, and by the late stages around 50 percent of patients exhibit at least some psychotic symptoms, with misidentification syndromes and hallucinations being more common in later stages.

Most psychotic symptoms can be successfully managed without the use of drugs if the patient is receiving constant care from a reliable caregiver. Many of the best interventions are discussed in chapter 4. The caregiver's role involves providing the person with constant reassurance, redirecting attention to other matters when delusions or hallucinations arise, and being compassionate and understanding when a patient misidentifies a person or object. People who are not responsive to these interventions may require treatment with what are known as neuroleptic or antipsychotic medications (see appendix B). High-potency neuroleptics including haloperidol (Haldol®) and fluphenazine (Prolixin®) are often the drugs of choice because they have relatively few uncomfortable side effects, although they may cause muscle spasms, facial tics, or stiffness of the limbs. A newer agent called risperidone

(Risperdal®) may have even fewer side effects but has not yet been used extensively in people with Alzheimer's disease. If given at low doses (e.g., 0.5 to 1 mg Haldol once or twice daily), these high-potency neuroleptics may be useful and relatively safe for someone with Alzheimer's disease. Low-potency antipsychotics (such as chlorpromazine [Thorazine®]) and thioridazine [Mellaril®]) are less desirable for use in elderly populations, because they can have potentially serious side effects, including low blood pressure and heart rhythm irregularities. Low blood pressure (also called hypotension) is of particular concern, because it often causes dizziness or lightheadedness and can lead to falls or fractures, which are difficult for older people to recover from.

TREATMENT OF COGNITIVE CHANGES

The drug hydergine is often prescribed for the treatment of cognitive changes in persons with Alzheimer's disease. Although it has demonstrated no more than limited success in improving a patient's cognition, mood, or ability to participate in normal activities, it has few side effects and has been given for many years, especially because there were no alternatives until recently.

In 1993 the Food and Drug Administration (FDA) approved the marketing of tacrine (Cognex®), still the only drug available in the United States that treats the cognitive decline associated specifically with Alzheimer's disease. Although results are not completely consistent, it appears that tacrine may be of limited benefit for perhaps up to 40 percent of those people who take it, particularly those who are in good physical health with mild-to-moderate cognitive symptoms. The benefits have been likened to the reversal of the deterioration of the patient's past 6 to 12 months, with improvement in communication, initiative, and sociability being somewhat greater than improvement in memory. Patients do continue deteriorating, however, and tacrine does not appear to slow the rate of disease progression beyond the initial 6-to-12 month reversal. It is difficult to determine what the improvement is worth, given that tacrine is quite expensive (about $100 a month), and that 15 percent or more of patients experience nausea, with another 30 to 50 percent experiencing liver damage. Though this damage is reversible, the potential complications make weekly liver function tests a costly and inconvenient necessity for approximately the first 6 months of treatment. Also, side effects prevent many people from tolerating a dosage of tacrine that would be high enough to be beneficial. Despite its shortcomings, many families are willing to try tacrine in the hopes that it will alleviate at least some of the cognitive deterioration seen in patients. The availability of tacrine has in any case opened the door to renewed drug development in the area of Alzheimer's disease, a benefit which, in time, should yield effective treatments.

Over-the-counter treatments

Health food stores and pharmacies may carry over-the-counter treatments that some people claim help to relieve some of the symptoms of Alzheimer's disease. Some are touted as "cognitive enhancers" or "smart drugs," and others are simple herbs advertised as "natural" treatments. A good number of these treatments are imported from or were originally developed in countries—China and India, in particular—where medicine is practiced differently from how it is in the United States. From a Western medical standpoint, some of these treatments contain potent chemicals (derived from natural sources, usually) that could be dangerous if used over a long period of time, while ingredients in other treatments may have no known effect on humans. Other treatments are based on Western medical theories, but most have not been tested rigorously, and none is endorsed by the FDA. Often there is a plausible rationale for the development of these treatments. For example, some studies have shown that

Alzheimer's disease patients suffer a deficiency of vitamin B12, so a potential treatment could be vitamin B12 supplements. But there is no evidence that the B12 deficiency is relevant to the symptoms of Alzheimer's disease; it may just be an incidental consequence of the disease. It is impossible to tell whether this treatment is helpful, because it has not been rigorously tested. Similarly, lecithin was at one time believed to have potential as a treatment for Alzheimer's disease. Although research has shown that this is not the case, lecithin is still available in health food stores. We recommend that a patient wanting to try an unproven therapy do so in the context of a scientifically monitored clinical trial (see chapter 6) that can prove or disprove the validity of the therapy, as well as providing careful monitoring of possible side effects. Obviously it is important for a patient and/or caregiver to discuss any proposed treatment with a doctor first.

6. Searching for a Cure

HOW RESEARCH IS CONDUCTED

Although tacrine is the only drug currently available in the United States for the treatment of the cognitive effects of Alzheimer's disease, current research suggests that it may not be long before there are more. Investigators are working to develop compounds that can alleviate the symptoms of Alzheimer's disease, slow or halt the disease once it has been diagnosed, or even prevent the disease entirely. Before looking at the various avenues of research that present possibilities, both of improving diagnosis of Alzheimer's disease and of developing treatments for it, we will discuss the drug development process in general in order to illustrate the hurdles a drug must clear before it can be marketed in the United States.

Understanding the drug development process is worthwhile for people with Alzheimer's disease and their families for several reasons. Anyone with Alzheimer's disease may be asked to participate in research studies, and because there are so few readily available treatments, patients may well benefit from participation. Furthermore, because dementia lessens a patient's competence to ask the right questions about a particular research study, families or caregivers are often required to participate in making decisions regarding consent to participate. It is wise for patients and families to discuss these issues early in the course of disease when patients can still understand them.

The process of drug development is both expensive and lengthy. According to the Pharmaceutical Manufacturers Association of the United States, it costs a pharmaceutical company an average of $359 million and takes 12 years to get one new compound from the laboratory to the pharmacy. Despite recent efforts to streamline this process, especially for drugs designed to treat some of the most visible serious diseases, including cancer, AIDS, and Alzheimer's disease, the length of time needed to develop a new drug is not likely to shrink substantially in the foreseeable future.

Any new compound being developed as a treatment for Alzheimer's disease has to go through several stages of testing before it can be marketed. The first stage is *preclinical* (*clinical* describes any procedure performed on humans). In the preclinical stage, drugs are tested in various models thought to represent the disease process. Investigators may examine the effect of the drug first in tissue samples or cell cultures in order to determine, for example, whether or not the drug affects the type of cell it has been designed for. Later, tests are performed on live animals. Some animal studies analyze the safety of the drug, looking for patterns of toxicity in animals to identify potentially dangerous compounds and prevent their use in humans. Other animal studies look for evidence that the drug will have the desired effect, which can be tricky when developing drugs for Alzheimer's disease because animals don't actually get the disease. Aged rodents and monkeys are sometimes used because they display cognitive losses similar to those seen in humans, even though the losses do not appear to have the same causes as those in Alzheimer's disease.

Scientists continue to look for better ways to predict the effectiveness of compounds through animal studies. Recently a team of researchers genetically engineered a strain of mice that develop amyloid plaques and lose synapses in areas of the brain affected by Alzheimer's disease. Such mice are called *transgenic* mice, because to create them a gene is *transferred* from another species. In this case, the transferred gene—or *transgene*—was the APP gene with the particular mutation found to cause early-onset familial Alzheimer's disease in humans (see chapter 3). The mutated

gene, packaged with genetic material that encourages it to
become active in the mouse, is injected into mouse eggs,
which are then fertilized and implanted in a female mouse.
The offspring that show evidence of successfully incorpo-
rating the inserted gene are then bred, and their offspring
are examined for signs of Alzheimer's disease. While it is
clear that the brains of these transgenic mice show features
common in Alzheimer's disease, it is yet unknown whether
these animals will also have behavioral or cognitive problems
resembling the deficits seen in the disease. After all, the mice
have only one of the problems associated with Alzheimer's
disease—overproduction of beta amyloid—and other disease
characteristics, such as neurofibrillary tangles or synapse loss
in general, may turn out to be more important. Nevertheless,
these mice may prove to be helpful in testing the worth of
treatments designed to halt the formation of plaques from
beta amyloid.

After preclinical studies have been completed and the
company developing the compound has gotten permission
from the FDA to test the drug in humans, the compound
goes through three phases of clinical testing. Phase I studies
test the safety of the investigational drug in a small number
of young healthy volunteers and, often, a small number of
healthy elderly volunteers, and determine what dose will
be best tolerated in patients. Phase II studies look at the
effectiveness of the drug in people with Alzheimer's disease
and the range of side effects that is possible. Phase III studies
test the drug in large groups of Alzheimer's disease patients
in order to verify effectiveness and determine whether any
side effects result from long-term use. If the compound shows
good results in Phase III studies, the company that developed
it then submits a new drug application to the FDA. This
document, running 100,000 pages or more, requests approval
to market a new drug and typically contains all of the known
data on it. Once various FDA committees have had a chance
to examine the data, a decision is reached.

With tacrine, this process took longer than usual. Because liver damage was common and benefits seemed marginal, tacrine was not approved when its maker originally submitted a new drug application in 1991. Further studies were conducted in larger groups of patients over a longer period of time to permit more detailed assessment of tacrine's effect on the liver, and data from these studies persuaded the FDA to approve the drug in 1993. Fortunately, pharmaceutical companies have learned from the development of tacrine and have been able to adjust the development plan for other drugs being developed for Alzheimer's disease to reduce the overall development time.

When trying to decide whether or not to participate in a research study for Alzheimer's disease, families should consider a number of issues. One important concern will be what organizations are conducting and sponsoring the study. Most projects are supported by foundations, government programs, or pharmaceutical companies and are carried out by universities, hospitals, and private doctors and medical groups. All must be reviewed by either a human subjects committee or an institutional review board, groups of doctors and lay people from a wide range of disciplines who evaluate studies to make sure that they are ethically sound and that the benefits of participating outweigh any potential risks to patients.

Another important concern is the design of the study itself. Families should understand what question the study is trying to answer and how the study design will help the investigators answer it. Most studies that involve the testing of investigational drugs use a relatively standard design, which makes it possible to compare one study to another. Following are some of the basic principles of research design. These may be considered in the evaluation of a forthcoming study or of results that have been reported in the news.

A basic element of clinical studies is placebo control. In a placebo-controlled study, typically one-fourth to one-half of the subjects are given placebos—capsules or tablets that look just like the investigational drug but that contain an inactive substance instead of the actual compound. Usually a computer program using random numbers determines which patients get which treatment. A placebo group serves as a comparison group that did not receive the drug but was otherwise treated exactly the same.

Good studies will also be double-blind—that is, neither the patient nor the persons responsible for treatment will know whether a patient is receiving placebo or drug. Someone associated with the sponsoring pharmaceutical company holds that information in coded form, but no one looks at it until the study is over and data are being analyzed. This additional precaution helps to control for a factor known as the *placebo effect*. In most clinical studies, most participants improve at least a little regardless of whether they are receiving placebo or the investigational drug. These improvements, or placebo effects, are generally considered to be results of receiving attention from a concerned physician, perhaps in a well-known medical clinic, of feeling important and proud to be participating in a research study, and of simply expecting to improve. Studies have shown that the expectations of patients and doctors actually influence a patient's improvement, so that knowing what treatment a patient was receiving could cause the doctor to behave in subtle ways that might change the patient's outcome. Keeping this information secret ensures that investigators will treat people who receive an investigational drug exactly the same as people who receive placebo. The investigators can thus determine whether any improvements in the people who are receiving the drug being tested can be attributed to that drug rather than to the placebo effect.

The placebo group is indispensable in allowing researchers to untangle what is actually happening in a study. If everyone in a study receives the drug and improves, it is impossible to tell whether the improvement was caused by the drug or by nonspecific placebo effects. However, if a placebo group is used, investigators know that any improvement in the drug group *beyond* what is seen in the placebo group can probably be attributed to the drug. Also, the timing at which any improvements appear and whether or not they are persistent compared to improvements in the placebo group provide important information for investigators.

Some people are unwilling to participate in placebo-controlled studies because they would rather know that they are receiving an active treatment that could potentially improve their condition. Remember, however, that placebo-controlled trials are the most important indicators of a treatment's worth. Patients can be proud to be part of the latest research, and they are generally assured of free high-quality care and treatment during the trials. After participating in a placebo-controlled study, patients are sometimes given the option to receive treatment with the investigational drug without placebo. This is generally referred to as a "compassionate" treatment since research is not the primary goal, although the information gained, particularly long-term safety information, may still be useful. The availability of this option generally depends on how far along in development a compound is and how beneficial it appears to be.

Clinical Trials in Alzheimer's Disease: Special Problems

There are some aspects of Alzheimer's disease that make the study of treatments difficult. Diagnosis is perhaps the most significant of these issues. In tests of drugs designed to reduce blood pressure, for example, it is relatively easy to be sure that those in the study actually have high blood pressure. But it is difficult to be certain that people with probable Alzheimer's disease actually have it. They might have, for example, Pick's disease or multi-infarct dementia, diseases that could respond differently to experimental treatments than would Alzheimer's disease. Therefore potential participants must be carefully screened to increase certainty that all the subjects in a research project have probable Alzheimer's disease. These screening procedures are often lengthy but provide an excellent work-up for diagnosis and on occasion may reveal another reason for the memory loss.

Another issue involves measuring improvement. At this time the majority of studies evaluating the merit of new treatments administer neuropsychological tests to subjects before and after treatment, looking for improvement in test scores or simply an absence of deterioration in scores, since the scores of untreated people can be expected to deteriorate over time (these studies typically run three or more months). Many neuropsychological tests, however, are influenced by factors such as previous administration, time of day, and mood of the patient as well as of the examiner, and may not reflect true mental capacities. Perhaps more important, even when mental test scores do not change or when they deteriorate, some treatments may help to alleviate other, more behavioral, symptoms of the disease, such as agitation, and this may improve the quality of life for patients even when the disease continues to progress.

Another difficulty with clinical trials in Alzheimer's disease is that, because they are invariably conducted in people who are generally healthy (other than having Alzheimer's disease), the results may not accurately reflect what would happen in an actual population of people with Alzheimer's disease. Elderly people frequently have chronic medical conditions such as high blood pressure, atherosclerosis, osteoarthritis, diabetes, osteoporosis, stroke, or cancer, most of which require regular medication. Furthermore, elderly people tend to be more sensitive than younger people to the effects of drugs, and the risk of negative side effects increases exponentially when more than one drug is taken at the same time. This could mean that an Alzheimer's drug that was well tolerated in a study population would not be as well tolerated by a real population of Alzheimer's patients who must also take drugs for other conditions. Nevertheless, clinical trials are conducted in healthy people in order to separate the effects of the drug being studied from the secondary effects of any other medications being taken.

HOPE FOR THE FUTURE

Future Diagnostic Tools

A major goal of Alzheimer's research is to find a biological marker that would permit development of a simple lab test for the disease, something as simple as a pregnancy test that would accurately diagnose Alzheimer's disease early in the disease's progression. Because Alzheimer's disease is so difficult to diagnose, clinicians are often unsure of their diagnosis until the disease progresses to the moderate or severe stage, at which time treatment may be less helpful. Early diagnosis would maximize the usefulness of available treatment and enable people with Alzheimer's disease and their families to prepare adequately for future medical needs and make appropriate financial and legal decisions as early as possible in the course of disease. Several lines of research look promising.

As we saw in chapter 3, geneticists have found some evidence that at least some forms of Alzheimer's disease are caused by genetic mutations. People from families in which familial Alzheimer's disease is common may soon be able to undergo screening procedures to determine whether they have mutations in the gene known to cause Alzheimer's disease in their family. This procedure, however, will only be useful for a small percentage of people affected by Alzheimer's disease.

The study that showed that the APO E4 form of the apolipoprotein E gene increases risk for all types of Alzheimer's disease and that PET scans showed decreased brain activity in Alzheimer's patients and in people judged to be at risk for Alzheimer's has led to a great deal of hope that a useful genetic screen for Alzheimer's might be developed.

A diagnostic tool that could identify people at risk for developing Alzheimer's years in advance would represent a major step forward in Alzheimer's disease research. Many questions require answers, however, before these findings could become the backbone of a good diagnostic test. It is important to note, for example, that the APO E4 form of the gene is not particularly widespread in the population, that not all people who carry it get Alzheimer's disease, and that many people who do not carry an APO E4 gene *do* get Alzheimer's disease. Thus the use of such a diagnostic test would still be limited.[5] Furthermore, only a few laboratories are capable of determining what type of APO E genes any particular individual carries,[6] and PET scans are expensive and time-consuming. Considerable refinement of genetic testing and PET scanning procedures would be required to make this type of diagnostic procedure feasible for widespread use, if it is indeed determined to be valuable.

Another simpler potential test would distinguish people who have Alzheimer's disease from people who don't by examining how much a person's pupils dilate when given eye drops of a very dilute solution of tropicamide, a drug that is routinely used by eye doctors to dilate the pupils. The team of researchers who reported this test in late 1994[7] found that most normal people barely responded to the dilute solution, showing no or nearly no pupil dilation. Eighteen out of 19 people with Alzheimer's disease, however, showed pupil dilations of 13 percent or more. The investigators believe that Alzheimer's patients may be extra sensitive to drugs that block the effects of acetylcholine, a chemical in the brain that is made by the same neurons that degenerate in Alzheimer's disease (see discussion in chapter 3). Especially interesting was their finding that one person in the control (normal) group who showed a significant pupil dilation was later found to have symptoms of dementia, suggesting that the changes in the brain that cause Alzheimer's disease significantly precede the onset of symptoms. If their results can be confirmed in larger studies, this simple inexpensive test could prove extremely helpful in diagnosing people early in the course of disease.

Another possible avenue for a simple diagnostic test was suggested by a study that showed an abnormality in potassium channel functioning in Alzheimer's disease patients.[8] Potassium channels can be thought of as gateways in the membranes that control movement of various fluids and materials into and out of cells. The investigators in this study looked at potassium channels because they show changes during memory formation. They theorized that memory loss might be associated with changes in potassium channels. They further postulated that if Alzheimer's is a disease that ultimately involves all the systems in the body, then it is possible that any changes in potassium channel functioning might show up in cells throughout the body and not just in the neurons where memory acquisition is actually taking place. The investigators found that one particular type of potassium channel did not work in people with Alzheimer's disease. While this may or may not have any effect on the overall functioning of patients, if it is true it could provide a basis for developing a skin test for Alzheimer's disease much like the tuberculin skin test for tuberculosis.

A fourth strategy proposed as a possible diagnostic test is to measure levels of various substances in cerebrospinal fluid. This procedure, called a lumbar puncture (or more colloquially, a spinal tap), is done by inserting a needle into someone's spinal cord between two vertebrae of the lower back and drawing a small amount of fluid out. One group of investigators reported that the cerebrospinal fluid of Alzheimer's disease patients contained higher than normal levels of a chemical called homovanillic acid in response to infusion with arecoline, a drug that blocks the action of acetylcholine.[9] If this is confirmed, it is likely the result of a mechanism similar to that of the pupil dilation discussed above. A more recent (and more promising) series of studies found high levels of the protein tau in cerebrospinal fluid of people with Alzheimer's disease. Although tau's role in the formation of neurofibrillary tangles is becoming increasingly well understood, no one is sure why it might occur at high levels in the cerebrospinal fluid. Nevertheless, if these studies are confirmed, then cerebrospinal fluid measurements of tau may become a useful adjunct for diagnosis.

One problem with examining cerebrospinal fluid for particular substances is that lumbar punctures are quite uncomfortable and inconvenient; furthermore, they carry a risk of damage to the nervous system, either from infection or from the needle itself. Doctors prefer to perform them only when absolutely necessary; thus, investigators must verify that diagnosis will be significantly improved by use of the procedure before doctors will be comfortable making it a routine diagnostic tool.

Until a specific biological marker for Alzheimer's disease is found and a simple lab test developed, clinicians and researchers will continue to refine procedures for use of NINCDS-ADRDA and DSM-IV criteria, neuropsychological tests, and brain scanning techniques to maximize the accuracy of Alzheimer's disease diagnosis. Even if a lab test is devised, it will need to be tested for accuracy in a large number of people before being made available to the general public. All lab tests have what are known as false positive and false negative rates; in other words, a percentage of people who appear to have a disease or problem actually do not (false positive), and a percentage who appear to be disease- or problem-free do have the disease (false negative). It is important to know how high these rates are so that doctors and patients can know how certain to be of their lab results. In cases where lab tests are known to have high false negative rates, for example, doctors may wish to repeat tests that turn up negative, especially if the person's symptoms are all consistent with a particular diagnosis. Similarly, people who test positive for life-threatening diseases, such as human immunodeficiency virus (the virus that causes AIDS), are routinely given the lab test again, in case their result was a false positive. Although determining the false positive and false negative rates can slow down the process of bringing a diagnostic test to the public, it is a worthwhile endeavor.

Symptomatic Therapies

Generally, the majority of treatments tested so far have been designed to alleviate cognitive symptoms of Alzheimer's disease rather than cure the disease itself. A great number of these therapies have concentrated on the known link between deficits of the neurotransmitter acetylcholine and cognitive impairment, despite the lack of understanding of the causal relationship. The idea that mental functioning may be enhanced by bolstering the activity of the cholinergic system— the system of neurons that produce and use acetylcholine— is known as the *cholinergic hypothesis*. The theory assumes that increasing acetylcholine levels in the brain may at least partially compensate for the loss of neurons, permitting some measure of cognitive improvement. Some degree of support for the hypothesis comes from the finding that drugs known to disrupt the cholinergic system, such as scopolamine, can also disrupt memory and learning. Thus it is believed that drugs that enhance activity of the cholinergic system might *improve* memory and learning.

Early efforts to increase levels of acetylcholine in the cholinergic system involved providing large amounts of the chemicals that the body uses to make acetylcholine, particularly lecithin and choline, but this approach failed. A second strategy involves drugs known as *muscarinic receptor agonists*. Muscarinic receptors, found on nerve cells in various parts of the body, are a class of receptors that can be stimulated by acetylcholine. As you will recall from chapter 2, the binding of neurotransmitters or other similar chemicals to receptors causes the neuron to fire, sending an electrical message on to another neuron. A muscarinic receptor agonist, then, is any drug that binds to a muscarinic receptor and stimulates the firing of the host neuron (whereas a muscarinic receptor *antagonist* would be a drug that would bind and then inhibit the firing of the neuron). Artificially stimulating neurons that normally respond to acetylcholine could compensate for the deficit of acetylcholine seen in Alzheimer's disease and thus has the potential to improve cognitive functioning.

Early trials of muscarinic receptor agonists, including arecoline, bethanechol, and RS86, were largely unsuccessful because the side effects they caused at the dosages thought to be potentially useful were too uncomfortable for patients to tolerate. These side effects, including nausea and vomiting, diarrhea, sweating, and increased salivation, are often referred to as cholinergic side effects and are caused by stimulation of muscarinic receptors in parts of the body besides the brain. The past ten years has seen an explosion in knowledge of muscarinic receptors, and investigators have learned that there are five separate types. The three types of muscarinic receptors that have been best characterized are M_1, M_2, and M_3, and they can be found primarily in the brain, heart and blood vessels, and glandular systems, respectively, though some of each type of receptor may be found in any part of the body. Cholinergic side effects are especially common when M_2 or M_3 receptors—the muscarinic receptors *outside* the brain— are stimulated. Increased understanding of this relationship has led to the development of muscarinic receptor agonists that stimulate only one type of muscarinic receptor.

Targeting the M_1 receptor limits the unwanted side effects that are caused primarily by stimulation of M_2 and M_3 receptors. A good number of specific M_1 receptor agonists, including xanomeline tartrate, CI-979, PD142505, FKS508, YM796, L687306, and L689660, are currently being developed and tested in Alzheimer's disease patients. (Pharmaceutical companies generally assign number codes to drugs while the drugs are being tested; if a drug gets far into development

it will later be given a more standard name. Thus if any of
the above code-named drugs are ever marketed, it will most
likely be under a different name.) An encouraging study of
xanomeline tartrate at doses of 25, 50, and 75 mg three times
daily in approximately 300 patients showed some improvement on neuropsychological tests and behavioral measures in
the patients on the highest dose. Studies of xanomeline and
other compounds continue.

While these M1 receptor agonists are more selective for M1
receptors than for M2 or M3 receptors, they still stimulate M2
and/or M3 receptors to some degree at higher doses, so that
it remains difficult to achieve a dosage of drug that is high
enough to reverse cognitive deficits without also inducing side
effects. Nevertheless, investigators continue to search for a
truly selective M1 receptor agonist in order to get around this
problem.

A third strategy to increase the activity of the cholinergic
system makes use of acetylcholinesterase (AChE) inhibitors,
drugs that prolong the effects of natural acetylcholine by preventing the enzyme acetylcholinesterase from breaking down
acetylcholine. This class of drugs, which includes tacrine,
has shown the most consistent, if modest, ability to improve
cognition in people with Alzheimer's disease. The first AChE
inhibitor to be closely studied was physostigmine. In most
studies, patients showed better scores on neuropsychological
tests, although the improvements were so small that they were
not outwardly noticeable to observers. Improvement varied
tremendously from patient to patient and was generally of
short duration where it did occur. Furthermore, there was
very little margin between effective doses and those that
caused cholinergic side effects. Unlike M1-specific muscarinic
receptor agonists, AChE inhibitors operate on centrally located cholinergic neurons in the brain *and* on the cholinergic neurons in other parts of the body that make up the
peripheral cholinergic system. At high doses AChE inhibitors
stimulate peripheral cholinergic activity, leading to the same

kinds of cholinergic side effects—nausea and vomiting, diarrhea, sweating—seen when M2 or M3 muscarinic receptors
are stimulated. The problems with physostigmine prompted a
search for an AChE inhibitor that would have more universal
and longer-lasting positive effects and fewer negative effects.
Tacrine is the first drug resulting from this research that has
been approved. Its many drawbacks, however, as discussed
earlier in the chapter, include a lack of tolerance at the doses
necessary to produce a positive effect, and have kept investigators searching for better compounds. A number of AChE
inhibitors are currently being developed, including velnacrine,
eptastigmine, and SDZ ENA 713.

Other neurotransmitter systems besides the cholinergic
system are affected in Alzheimer's disease and may also be
appropriate targets for drug development. These include the
dopamine, serotonin, norepinephrine, and peptide systems.
There are already some drugs being tested that target more
than one neurotransmitter system, such as besipirdine, which
affects both the cholinergic and adrenergic systems.

Another strategy being developed to offer symptomatic
relief is the use of nootropics. These are psychoactive drugs
that stimulate brain mechanisms affecting cognitive performance by enhancing cerebral metabolism (use of energy by
the brain). Hydergine is an example of a nootropic already in
use, though whether it is truly effective is debatable. Other
nootropics, such as piracetam, are available in Europe, but
their efficacy is also uncertain. When nootropics are combined with cholinomimetics—a more general term for drugs
that affect the cholinergic system, including both muscarinic
agonists and AChE inhibitors—some Alzheimer's disease
patients have shown mild improvement in social behavior and
attention, though not in cognitive function.

Yet another symptomatic treatment for Alzheimer's disease is based on the finding that enzymes dependent on the
vitamin thiamine are decreased in the brain of Alzheimer's
disease patients. Thiamine itself is important in metabolism

and in cholinergic systems, in modulating cholinergic activity. One study of high doses of thiamine hydrochloride appeared to produce mild improvement in cognitive function. Some investigators feel this is due to a cholinergic effect of thiamine, since high-dose thiamine can partially reverse the adverse cognitive effects of the anticholinergic agent scopolamine. Most researchers do not believe thiamine treatment is a promising strategy, however, and therefore no long-term studies of its safety or efficacy have been performed.

Preventive Therapies

Hypotheses to explain how Alzheimer's disease comes about are still quite controversial. There is probably a variety of causes, many of them interrelated, which culminate in a single disease characterized by dementia and behavioral changes and associated with neuritic plaques, neurofibrillary tangles, and serious deficits in brain neurotransmitter systems. While this wide assortment of causes can be bewildering, the variety of theories means that research can be conducted along many paths, increasing the likelihood that one or more will lead to a useful treatment.

Since the dysfunction in patients with Alzheimer's disease is due to the loss of neurons and synapses, drugs that try to change the activity of neurotransmitters or improve brain metabolism are not likely to produce dramatic cognitive improvements or arrest the progression of the disease. Efforts to slow the deterioration of neurons, however, might be helpful. Thus investigators are trying to develop drugs that will prevent, arrest, or even reverse the biochemical events that lead to the cognitive deficits in Alzheimer's disease. Treatment ideas include neuroprotective drugs, which would protect existing neurons from damage, and neurotrophic drugs, which encourage continued sprouting of neurons that have been damaged. Another possibility is tissue replacement therapies, in which tissues that could produce the necessary chemical factors would be implanted, or corrected gene sequences could be spliced into the genes that code for proteins that cause problems. All of these strategies (particularly the tissue replacement ideas) are in the early stages of development, but significant progress has been made in recent years, and there is reason to believe that one or more of these ideas may result in a useful treatment.

Neuroprotective treatments— Therapies that center around preventing nerve damage and death represent an important direction for research. The finding that amyloid accumulation leads to nerve damage has prompted a number of creative approaches. As we saw in chapter 3, the amyloid precursor protein (APP) is normally cut down to produce soluble-APP, or, less often, the smaller protein beta amyloid. With Alzheimer's disease, however, a processing error leads to a decrease in production of soluble-APP and increase in beta amyloid. Soluble-APP appears to make neurons more resistant to certain types of nerve damage, and also seems to promote nerve growth. Beta amyloid, on the other hand, attaches to neurons and appears to cause cell death. Both genetic and environmental factors appear to influence this process.

One strategy for intervention would be to prevent the formation or accumulation of amyloid, which could be done by inhibiting the enzymes that cut APP to form beta amyloid. This has been shown to work in laboratory tests, and would reduce the burden of beta amyloid that neurons need to deal with. Another strategy would be to block the toxicity caused by beta amyloid once it has been formed. An agent that could stabilize cells and rescue them from amyloid-induced damage could be useful. One chemical known as Substance P may prevent damage caused by amyloid; however, there is no good way to deliver this substance to the brain, because it cannot cross the blood-brain barrier, a safety mechanism that prevents most potentially toxic substances in the bloodstream from entering the brain. Thus intravenous administration of Substance P would not work, and techniques to administer substances directly into the brain are quite difficult. Another chemical, a dye called Congo red, has been shown to inhibit the nerve damage amyloid causes by preventing the formation of new amyloid fibrils and binding to fibrils that are already there. More research will be necessary to determine whether an agent that could inhibit formation or toxicity of beta amyloid would have therapeutic value.

The toxicity of beta amyloid may be related to what are known as excitotoxic mechanisms. Excitatory chemicals are neurotransmitters that, when released into the synaptic cleft, *stimulate*, or excite, the receiving neuron. The most common excitatory neurotransmitter in the brain is the amino acid glutamate, which can stimulate several different types of receptors, including an important class known as NMDA receptors (named for their sensitivity to a chemical called N-methyl-D-aspartate). In normal neurotransmission, glutamate binds to receptors on the receiving neuron, which stimulates special channels in the cell's membrane to open so that calcium and other electrically charged molecules can flow in. The electric charge travels down the length of the neuron and stimulates the release of more neurotransmitters to continue the message. After glutamate has done its job on the original receiving neuron, it is taken back up by the original sending neuron. If it remains in the synaptic cleft for a prolonged amount of time, however, its continued stimulation of the receptors can become toxic and cause death to the neurons involved. This kind of death by overstimulation is known as excitotoxicity. A suggested mechanism for this cell death involves calcium channels, the cell membrane gateways that open to allow calcium into the neuron when glutamate receptors are stimulated. Overstimulation of glutamate receptors permits the channels to remain open for long periods of time, allowing higher than normal concentrations of calcium to build up within the cell. Prolonged exposure to calcium may lead to cell death.

Excitotoxicity is well established as a mechanism for neuronal death in a number of acute neurological diseases, including ischemia, trauma, anoxia, and epileptic seizures. It therefore might play a role in neurodegenerative diseases. One clue is that beta amyloid or fragments of it seem to have no neurotoxic effect when tested alone on brain tissue in the laboratory, but *have* been shown to promote neuronal death when glutamate is also present and behaving excitotoxically. Furthermore, a reduction in the number of sites for glutamate uptake has been noted in Alzheimer's disease, while rates of glutamate release and glutamate concentration seem to be normal. Investigators speculate that a decreased capacity to take glutamate back into the cell could result in receptors being exposed to glutamate for extended periods of time.

Two classes of drugs might prevent excitotoxic cell death. If calcium build-up is a major factor in this process, as some investigators speculate, then drugs known as calcium-channel blockers may be useful because they physically block calcium channels, preventing calcium from entering the neuron even when glutamate receptors are being stimulated. A second class of compounds that might be helpful are the NMDA antagonists. Neurons in different parts of the brain differ in their vulnerability to neuronal death through excitotoxicity, and stimulation of the NMDA subtype of glutamate receptor seems to trigger neuronal injury especially readily. NMDA antagonists prevent the stimulation of the NMDA subtype of glutamate receptor by physically blocking the site where glutamate would normally bind. Using an NMDA antagonist would prevent overstimulation of neurons, at least at the NMDA-subtype receptors, though glutamate would still be able to stimulate other types of glutamate receptors. Two NMDA antagonists that have already been studied are cycloserine and milacemide, neither of which was effective in Alzheimer's disease patients.

Another strategy for preventing the accumulation of beta amyloid involves an enzyme-inhibiting chemical called alpha-1-antichymotrypsin (ACT, sometimes written a_1-ACT) and the lipid transport protein apolipoprotein E (apoE). These have been found to be closely associated with beta amyloid in the filamentous amyloid deposits of Alzheimer's disease, and are thought to actually stimulate beta amyloid to form amyloid filaments, which then readily aggregate to form plaques. In one study, the form of apoE that has been linked to development of late-onset Alzheimer's disease—apoE4—had the greatest amyloid-promoting activity. Some investigators believe that amyloid plaques arise when beta amyloid is induced to form filaments by the presence of these amyloid-promoting factors in certain brain regions, which would explain why plaques do not form throughout the brain even though beta amyloid can occur anywhere. Steps in this process, including interactions between ACT and/or apoE and beta amyloid could serve as logical targets for intervention.

Another possible strategy might be to interrupt the formation of neurofibrillary tangles. As we saw in chapter 3, these lesions are made of tau proteins that have been hyperphosphorylated, meaning that several phosphorous and oxygen groups have bonded to the protein. Investigators have noted that in laboratory studies, apoE3 and apoE2 can bind to the tau proteins, whereas apoE4 cannot. Perhaps the interaction between apoE3 or E2 and tau proteins protects tau from hyperphosphorylation and in doing so prevents formation of neurofibrillary tangles. Furthermore, apoE can be involved in peripheral nerve regeneration after a lesion has developed; apoE3 plus a source of lipid helps neurites (the outermost projections of neurons) to grow and join up to compensate in areas where many neurons have died, whereas apoE4 inhibits this beneficial growth. The two forms therefore affect the ability of nerve cells to compensate for progression of disease differently. This could explain why people who carry the APO E4 gene appear to develop Alzheimer's disease

more often or at a younger age than those with APO E3 or
APO E2. A delay in age of onset might be induced by a drug
that behaved like apoE2 or E3 and prolonged the survival
of affected nerve cells. A search for such a compound has
already begun, while research into the mechanisms of action
of the different forms of apolipoprotein E continues.

Neurotrophic treatments— Neurotrophic substances promote the growth of neurons and neurites. For example, nerve
growth factor is one of several naturally occurring chemicals
that help neurites survive and regenerate and enhance neuronal function, at least in adult primates. Use of nerve growth
factor or factors like it might increase survival of diseased
neurons or restore activity to those that have become inactive.
In animals, nerve growth factor slows down the loss of cells
when an area of the brain called the *nucleus basalis of Meyn-
ert* is damaged (this area shows significant damage in people
with Alzheimer's disease). Nerve growth factors are hard to
work with, however; they do not reach the brain if they are
administered intravenously because of the blood-brain barrier.
Furthermore, there are only a few areas of the brain where
neurons respond to nerve growth factor, and no one knows
whether enough of the appropriate neurons are responsive for
nerve growth factor to be especially valuable. It is possible
that in the future, cells could be genetically engineered to
produce a neurotrophic factor that would induce response in
a larger variety of neuron types. If, in the future, doctors are
able to diagnose Alzheimer's disease even before symptoms
show up, administration of nerve growth factor or factors like
it might help to prevent nerve damage from progressing to
the point where patients start to show symptoms.

Another treatment related to nerve growth involves *gangliosides*. These substances play a role in neuronal plasticity,
the phenomenon in which neurons reestablish or rearrange
connections between neurons, even rebuilding their neurites.
This plasticity is only possible when the cell body receives

a continuous supply of appropriate nerve growth factors, proteins, and gangliosides. Gangliosides are required specifically for the branching out of neurites and the creation of new synapses where two neurites from different neurons come together. Both alone and in combination with nerve growth factor, gangliosides enhance neuron differentiation and outgrowth in tissue cultures, and, in rats and monkeys, ganglioside treatment reduces degeneration and shrinkage of neurons, and increases cholinesterase activity. It is not possible to determine whether the effects are due to the prevention of neurite loss or restoration of lost connections. Gangliosides have also been used, with limited success, as treatments in some cases of neural injury such as head trauma, spinal cord injury, and stroke.

Some studies have shown that there is a significant loss of gangliosides in those with Alzheimer's disease, particularly in the early-onset form. In one study gangliosides were administered via injection to 16 early Alzheimer's disease patients, and there was no sign of improvement. Because gangliosides, like nerve growth factors, cannot cross the blood-brain barrier, the same research group is in the midst of studying 10 patients who are being given gangliosides intracerebrally— that is, directly into their brains. This requires a surgical procedure in which thin tubes are implanted in spaces toward the front of the brain and attached to a small reservoir that is implanted in the scalp. Small tubes inserted under the skin attach the reservoir to a pump that is placed under the skin of the abdomen, where the fluid to be dispensed to the patient can be refilled once a month. Half the patients have been receiving this treatment for a year now, and in all five the disease process has been halted, psychiatric test scores have been unchanged or have improved, and patients are more active and well behaved. Although these results appear to be promising, the lack of a control group and double-blind conditions are troubling complications for reliable interpretation of results. Even if the apparent success can be confirmed, the complexity, invasiveness, and inconvenience of the drug delivery system for gangliosides are negative factors that require serious consideration.

Neural transplants— Some researchers are looking at the possibility of implanting neural tissue into the diseased brain. Such procedures are often referred to as neural transplants, even though the word *transplant* suggests that entire neurons are being replaced, as in a heart or liver transplant, which is not the case. A more accurate term is *neural graft*. In a neural graft, neural tissue from an external source is implanted into a brain and allowed to grow together with existing brain tissue.

In the brain and elsewhere in the nervous system, some types of neurons may atrophy or die if the neurons they are connected to are destroyed. Thus a few damaged neurons can set up a domino effect, resulting in greater damage than necessary. One experiment examined this effect in rats in which certain cholinergic neurons were deliberately damaged through excitotoxic mechanisms. Two approaches reversed the atrophy of the damaged neurons and allowed them to function again: injecting nerve growth factor, *or* injecting a suspension of fetal central nervous system tissue ground up into a liquid, into the ventricle of the brain. In another set of experiments in which lesions were induced in the cholinergic systems of rats, the implantation of intact rat fetal cholinergic neural tissue led to the restoration of normal motor and cognitive behaviors. The implanted neurons appear to substitute for original neurons by reconnecting to neurons whose connections had been lost, such that largely normal types of synaptic contacts are formed, and by restoring neurotransmitter release to normal or near-normal levels. Other experiments using aged rats instead of young or developing rats showed similar results. Importantly, these experiments show that the adult brain retains many of the mechanisms necessary to permit surviving neurons to establish new connections with other surviving or newly implanted neurons.

Neural grafting does seem to have potential to help repair neurons and allow them to work again in the damaged central nervous system. There are numerous problems with the technique, however, that must be resolved before it can be useful in the treatment of Alzheimer's disease. As we have seen, one significant problem is that animals do not get Alzheimer's disease, so that testing in animals does not give a wholly accurate picture of how the procedure might work in humans. Given the extreme invasiveness of any sort of implantation procedure, it would be valuable to know how well the procedure works in primates before testing the procedure in humans.

Similar concerns came up with an intracerebral cell implantation technique that has been tested (with some success) in people with Parkinson's disease. After success in a rat model, investigators went ahead and initiated clinical trials in Parkinson's patients without having tested the procedures in nonhuman primates, because there was no good Parkinson's disease model available in primates. Some controversy surrounded this research, and several investigators have recommended that similar studies in Alzheimer's disease patients be delayed if at all possible until an appropriate model for Alzheimer's disease in nonhuman primates can be developed.

It will also be difficult to select patients that are appropriate for use in clinical trials, and, later, for the procedures in general. At this time, grafting requires at least one major surgery with significant potential for complications, especially in an elderly population, so only patients in the best of health could be permitted to undergo the procedure. All procedures would have to be streamlined to increase safety before neural grafting could be tested in clinical trials in Alzheimer's disease patients, and improvement would have to be significant and long-lasting for this to become a routinely accepted treatment.

A third major problem involves ethics. It is still too early to say whether neural grafting will result in repair or reversal of the ravages of Alzheimer's disease. But if it does, chances are good that it will do so using neural tissues taken from human fetuses. Fetal tissue is preferable to tissue from other sources because its cells multiply faster, making recovery more rapid. It is also more likely to integrate easily into the host brain, because it doesn't contain the immune system components that would cause most other tissues to be recognized as foreign and be rejected. The main source of human fetal tissue, however, were it to be established as an effective transplant organ, is likely to be elective abortions—and therein lies the controversy.

Many people who find elective abortion immoral argue that any use of fetal tissue is also immoral, simply compounding the wrong being done to the fetus. They also object to the procedure because they believe that use of fetal tissue will change abortion practices in undesirable ways. In order to donate tissue, women might abort fetuses they might otherwise have carried to term; there could even be a resulting black market offering financial incentives to such women. Elective abortions might increase as a result, and might be legitimized by the perceived selflessness associated with tissue donation, so that the overturning of current laws permitting abortion would be less likely. Proponents of fetal tissue research, on the other hand, argue that certain legal measures could minimize incentives to abort. For example, they recommend not letting a woman name a recipient for any tissue she donates (unlike in most other types of organ/tissue donations, there is no evidence that a genetic similarity between the donor and recipient increases the success of fetal tissue transplants). They further recommend passing laws to forbid paying women for tissue donation and to prohibit abortion providers from asking a woman whether she would be willing to donate fetal tissue until she has already decided to have an abortion.

These issues are complex, and the controversy is not likely to disappear any time soon. Medical science may find sources of tissue for neural grafts that do not raise these thorny ethical questions: cell biology and genetic engineering techniques might allow the use of neural tissue from other parts of the recipient's own brain or genetically engineered tissue grown from human brain cells that would secrete particular useful factors (e.g., a generalized version of nerve growth factor or specific neurotransmitters). Furthermore, successful treatments derived from other areas of research may become available before grafting does. Any treatment that would not require a potentially dangerous major surgery would be infinitely preferable for its obvious advantages in terms of cost, safety and availability.

Other potential treatments— Women who use estrogen replacement therapy after menopause are less likely to develop Alzheimer's disease than women who do not. Several small studies have shown that estrogen replacement therapy has a positive effect on cognition in both cognitively impaired and normal postmenopausal women. Furthermore, estrogens have been shown to serve a maintenance role in the regions of the brain that are most affected in Alzheimer's disease, and they participate in the processing of both APP and apoE. If, indeed, estrogens play an important role in normal brain functioning, then it would stand to reason that estrogen replacement therapy could be helpful in postmenopausal women who no longer produce natural estrogen. (Why are men not affected? Throughout their lives, men produce testosterone, a hormone related to estrogen that can be converted to estrogen in the necessary areas of the brain.) Many investigators have suggested that large clinical trials of estrogens should be instituted. These could be initiated relatively easily since there is already available a variety of estrogen preparations with which the medical community has a great deal of experience.

Researchers are also investigating the role of the immune system in contributing to the symptoms of Alzheimer's disease. Alzheimer's disease is clearly not a traditional inflammatory disease, i.e., a disease that involves swelling and often pain due to local reactions of the immune system (the best known probably being arthritis). An elevation of immune system proteins in the brains of people with Alzheimer's disease, however, indicates that there is an active inflammatory response, often associated with amyloid plaques. Because these proteins are so frequently seen in conjunction with the disease, some people have hypothesized that anti-inflammatory medications, which can reduce the activity of these proteins, might be of use in treating Alzheimer's disease, although no one is sure what role the proteins might play in causing symptoms. Indeed, several retrospective studies have shown that people who regularly take nonsteroidal anti-inflammatory drugs for arthritis or rheumatism are somewhat less likely to develop Alzheimer's disease than people the same age who don't.

If immune system components—such as cytokines, found to exist at elevated levels in the brains of people with Alzheimer's disease—and immune activation in general cause or contribute to the pathology of Alzheimer's disease, drugs that could regulate the genes controlling inflammatory response might be useful. Genes that code for anti-inflammatory proteins could be stimulated to produce more protein, whereas genes that code for proteins causing inflammation could be inhibited. Furthermore, blockading the neural receptors that cytokines act upon could be a useful strategy if an effective agent could be found. The simplest strategy studied so far, however, has been the testing of indomethacin, a nonsteroidal anti-inflammatory drug widely used to treat arthritis. Encouraging results in small pilot studies have led to the initiation of larger clinical trials. An intervention based on the inflammatory response or other immune-mediated processes may prove to be a useful approach, either alone or in combination with other treatments.

Further research on the genetics of Alzheimer's disease may help in the search for a treatment. Defective genes that cause particular diseases can be used to develop animal models for the study of such diseases. With the application of complicated genetic techniques, the abnormal human gene is placed into the animal. If it is a good animal model, the transgenic animal will develop the same disease that humans develop (or something very similar), making that animal useful for testing treatments. Of course, genes that are known to cause disease in humans don't always cause disease in animals, which complicates development of a good animal model. But each gene that is discovered to be related to Alzheimer's disease has the potential to become useful in an animal model. Furthermore, since the genes that are involved all have different functions, each one controlling a distinct protein and each causing Alzheimer's disease through its own mechanism, each new gene that is found reveals a new potential target for therapy.

Everything known about Alzheimer's disease to date suggests that changes in the brain begin long before symptoms arise. This means that there is a large window of opportunity for treating Alzheimer's disease early *if* we can find a way to identify the people who are most at risk. It is possible that an untangling of the genetic causes of Alzheimer's disease may help in the development of genetic tests. These could not only identify which people are at risk but also the genes that put them at risk. If it is found that people with different genetic risk factors respond differently to each defect, treatment could involve an intervention tailored to a person's particular genetic defect.

There may be no "cure" for Alzheimer's disease, no treatment that would completely eradicate any evidence that the disease was ever present. However, it seems reasonable to think that there may someday be a treatment or treatments that will prevent potential Alzheimer's disease patients from ever experiencing the symptoms of dementia. Treatment of this nature will probably require an intervention that stops or prevents neuron death and the loss of synaptic networks as early as possible. But until something like this is developed and made available, symptomatic therapies may be the best

that can be offered. Fortunately there are 15 or 20 symptomatic therapies being tested in people with Alzheimer's disease in clinical trials right now; we can hope that at least one
will alleviate cognitive deficits and perhaps slow progression
of the disease.

Appendix A: NINCDS-ADRDA and DSM-IV Criteria for Alzheimer's Disease

NINCDS-ADRDA criteria for probable Alzheimer's disease	*DSM-IV criteria for Alzheimer's disease*
Probable Alzheimer's disease may be indicated by:	Alzheimer's disease is suggested by:

A. Clinically documented dementia
B. Progressive worsening of memory and other cognitive functions
C. Deficits in two or more cognitive areas
D. Onset between ages 40 and 90
E. Absence of systemic or brain disorders that could account for deficits
	A. Development of multiple cognitive deficits:
	  1. Memory impairment
	  2. Progressive deficits in language, motor skills, perception, or higher-order reasoning skills

Probable Alzheimer's disease is supported by: A. Progressive deficits in language (aphasia), motor skills (apraxia), and perception (agnosia) B. Impaired ability to function in everyday activities C. Family history of similar disorder D. Consistent lab results, such as CT scan showing cerebral atrophy	B. Continued gradual cognitive function decline C. Deficits interfering significantly with occupational and social functioning D. Exclusion of other causes of dementia
(Source: McKhann et al., 1984)	(Source: American Psychiatric Association, 1994)

American Psychiatric Association. *DSM-IV: Diagnostic and Statistical Manual of Mental Disorders*. 4th ed. Washington, D. C.: American Psychiatric Association, 1994.

McKhann, G., D. Drachman, M. Folstein, et al. "Clinical Diagnosis of Alzheimer's Disease: Report of the NINCDS-ADRDA Work Group." *Neurology* 34 (1984): 939–44.

Appendix B: Drug Treatments in Alzheimer's Disease

Symptom	Drugs	Comments
Depression	Fluoxetine HCl (Prozac); Sertraline HCl (Zoloft); Paroxetine HCl (Paxil)	These compounds, part of a class of drugs called selective serotonin reuptake inhibitors (SSRIs), may cause headache, nausea, or anxiety, but side effects are relatively minimal. They are nontoxic in overdose and may calm agitated patients without sedating.
	Nortriptyline HCl (Aventyl, Pamelor); Desipramine (Norpramin, Pertofrane)	Tricyclic antidepressants that may cause lightheadedness, dizziness, nausea, and sedation, but these effects are generally low-grade and well tolerated.
	Amitriptyline HCl (Elaril); Imipramine (Tofraril); Doxepine (Sinequan)	These tricyclic antidepressants often cause sedation, dizziness, and other cardiovascular effects in the elderly.
	Venlafaxine HCl (Effexor)	May cause nausea, nervousness or high blood pressure.
	Selegiline HCl (Eldepryl)	Some physicians recommend this anti-parkinson agent with antidepressant effects for its additional antioxidant effects.
	Bupropion HCl (Wellbutrin)	This compound is often good for lethargic patients, but may cause agitation, insomnia, nausea, and constipation.

Continued

Symptom	Drugs	Comments
Anxiety and agitation	Alprazolam (Xanax); Lorazepam (Ativan)	These compounds are part of the class of drugs known as benzodiazepines, which have some sedating effects. These two particular drugs have a shorter duration of action than other benzodiazepines, which is useful since prolonged sedation is not usually beneficial to the patient.
	Haloperidol (Haldol); Fluphenazine (Prolixin)	These drugs are high-potency neuroleptics, a general class of drugs designed for reducing symptoms of psychosis. This type of drug is recommended for use in Alzheimer's disease because there are fewer side effects than in the lower-potency agents, which are commonly associated with sedation, lightheadedness, and other uncomfortable symptoms. The high-potency drugs, however, may cause involuntary muscle spasms, facial tics, etc.
	Buspirone (Buspar)	This agent, an azapirone, is often useful for reducing symptoms of anxiety without inducing sedation. Common side effects include dizziness, insomnia, and nausea.
Paranoia	Haloperidol (Haldol)	Use only if the patient is unduly distressed and unresponsive to reassurances by the caregiver.

Continued

Symptom	Drugs	Comments
Hallucinations and/or delusions	Haloperidol (Haldol); Fluphenazine (Prolixin); Risperidone (Risperdal); Thioridazine (Mellaril)	Use drug treatment only if hallucinations seem to frighten the patient or result in bizarre or dangerous behavior.
Cognitive changes	Hydergine (Hydergine)	Hydergine has only limited benefits, but because it has few side effects is often tried. It should not be used if any psychoses are present.
	Tacrine HCl (Cognex)	Because tacrine has the potential to cause serious liver damage, liver function must be monitored regularly. Other possible side effects include nausea and/or vomiting, diarrhea, and abdominal pain. However, some patients with mild to moderate symptoms can benefit from treatment.

Appendix C: Suggestions for Further Reading/Viewing

PUBLICATIONS

The 36-Hour Day: A Family Guide to Caring for Persons with Alzheimer's Disease and Related Dementing Illnesses. Long considered the Bible of dementia caregiving, this landmark book is a must for every caregiver. Nancy L. Mace and Peter V. Rabins, Baltimore: Johns Hopkins University Press, 1991 (revised edition).

Understanding Alzheimer's Disease. Published by the Alzheimer's Disease and Related Disorders Association and edited by Miriam K. Aronson, this book is an outstanding review of Alzheimer's disease for the layperson. New York: Charles Scribner's Sons, 1988.

Homes That Help: Advice from Caregivers for Creating a Supportive Home for People with Alzheimer's. This incredible book is a wealth of information gathered from 90 experienced caregivers about how to create a comfortable and safe environment for a person with Alzheimer's. Richard Olsen, Ezra Ehrenkrantz, and Barbara Hutchings, Newark, N. J.: New Jersey Institute of Technology Press, 1993.

Alzheimer's: A Caregiver's Guide and Sourcebook. This book is another comprehensive source that describes what to expect in Alzheimer's disease and how to cope with its demands. Single copies of the book are available free of charge from the American Health Assistance Foundation (800-437-2433), or you can find it in bookstores. H. Gruetzner, John Wiley & Sons, 1992.

Rush Manual for Caregivers. This manual from the Rush Alzheimer's Disease Center in Chicago gives an overview of the issues that families of Alzheimer's patients face and provides guidelines for patient care. Available from the Rush Alzheimer's Disease Center (312-942-4463).

Alzheimer's Disease and Related Disorders Association
brochures include:
  Alzheimer's Disease: Services You May Need (1990)
  Caregiving at Home (1990)
  Communicating with the Alzheimer Patient (1990)
  Especially for the Alzheimer Caregiver (1990)
  Financial and Health Care You May Need (1991)
  Home Care with the Alzheimer's Patient (1988)
  Legal Considerations for Alzheimer's Patients (1991)
  Standing By You: Family Support Groups (1990)

Most chapters of the Alzheimer's Association publish newsletters which provide valuable information on current research and public policy and local events/support services that may be helpful.

Burke Rehabilitation Hospital Auxiliary, White Plains, N.Y., brochures:
  Home Management of the Person with Intellectual Loss
      (Dementia or Alzheimer's Disease) (1991)
  Choosing a Nursing Home for the Person with Intellectual
      Loss (1989)

*Care of Alzheimer's Patients: A Manual for Nursing Home
    Staff.* Although this manual was written especially for
    nursing home staff, home caregivers may find it useful
    too. Lisa Gwyther, Durham, N.C.: American Health Care
    Association and Alzheimer's Disease and Related Disor-
    ders Association, 1985.
Alzheimer's Disease: Optimizing Drug Development Strategies.
    This review of the issues involved in finding cures for
    Alzheimer's disease is appropriate for the more inter-
    ested reader. Neal R. Cutler, John J. Sramek, and Amy
    E. Veroff, Sussex, England: John Wiley & Sons, Ltd,
    1994.
How and Why We Age. Leonard Hayflick's bestseller is an
    extremely accessible and interesting book on aging in
    general. New York: Ballantine Books, 1994.

In addition, you may want to look for books from Elder Books, a small press dedicated to publishing practical, hands-on guidebooks for family and professional caregivers of people with Alzheimer's disease.

VIDEO/FILM

Quite a few videos have been produced about Alzheimer's disease; some deal with the emotional difficulties of caring for someone with the disease, while others discuss the search for a cure. Many of the videos listed below have appeared on television—usually public or cable stations—and you may be able to borrow copies from your local Alzheimer's Association chapter.

Complaints of a Dutiful Daughter. This Oscar-nominated film was shown on the acclaimed PBS program *Point of View* ("Independent Points of View from America's Independent Filmmakers") in 1994. It was produced, written, and directed by Deborah Hoffmann, who documents her experience with her mother's Alzheimer's disease. It can be ordered from Women Make Movies at 212-925-0606 for $275.

Something Must Be Done About Grandma Ruthie. AudioVisual Communications, The University of Chicago Medical Center, 1993.

Losing It All: The Reality of Alzheimer's Disease. Produced, written, and directed by Michael Mierendorf for HBO in 1991.

The Road to Galveston. U. S. A. Pictures, USA Cable TV, 1996 Wilshire Court Productions, Houston Film Commission. Supported by Rick Ferguson, Drew Mayer-Oakes and Peggy Lee of Coldsprings, Tex., and distributed by CNM Entertainment, Inc.

"Waves of Stone." Episode of *Medicine 2000* on Alzheimer's disease. Produced and directed by Dita Domonkos and

Lee R. Bobker for Vision Associates 1994, South Carolina
ETV. The program was made possible by the Research
and Medicine Division of Glaxo.

"The Behaving Brain" and "Remembering and Forgetting."
Episodes of *Discovering Psychology* on the Discovery
Channel, both with Philip Zimbardo, Ph.D., Stanford
University. Both programs were 1989 productions of
WGBH Boston, sponsored by the WGBH Educational
Foundation.

The Brain: Our Universe Within. This was a 5-part series
done by the Discovery Channel, with hour-long segments
called "Evolution," "Perception," "Memory," "Miraculous
Mind," and "Matter Over Mind." The third section deals
with Alzheimer's disease. A 1994 production of NHK,
NHK Creative, Inc., and Discovery Productions. The
whole series may be ordered from The Discovery Channel
at 1-800-587-1818 for $49.95, but, again, you may be able to
borrow copies from the Alzheimer's Association.

Future Quest "Designer Genes." A program on Alzheimer
gene research hosted by Jeff Goldblum. A 1994 production of Producer Entertainment Group supported by the
Corporation for Public Broadcasting.

Appendix D: Sources for Information and Support

The Alzheimer's Association, more formally known as the Alzheimer's Disease and Related Disorders Association (ADRDA), supports research on Alzheimer's disease and other similar disorders and provides support and assistance to patients and their families and caregivers. To find the chapter nearest you, order books or brochures, or learn more about the association and its programs, write to P.O. Box 5675, Chicago, Illinois 60680; phone 1-800-272-3900 (TDD: 312-335-8882); or fax 312-335-1110.

The Benjamin B. Green-Field National Alzheimer's Library and Resource Center is maintained out of the Alzheimer's Association Chicago offices. They may be reached at (312) 335-3602; or by e-mail at greenfld@class.org.

The National Institute on Aging, part of the National Institutes of Health, sponsors a great deal of research on Alzheimer's disease. Twenty-eight major medical institutions are NIA centers for diagnosis. The NIA set up the *Alzheimer's Disease Education and Referral Center (ADEAR)* as a clearinghouse for information on Alzheimer's disease. "Information specialists" at the center can help you find answers to just about any question you may have, and if they don't have the answers, they can direct you to people who do. They also provide listings of publications, videos, and support organizations, information on drug testing and clinical trials, information on the disease itself, and the latest in research findings. You can write the center at P.O. Box 8250, Silver Spring, Maryland 20907-8250; fax them at 301-587-4352; phone toll-free at 1-800-438-4380; or send e-mail to adear@alzheimers.org.

The Alliance for Aging Research is a nonprofit advocacy organization that works to increase the priority of research on aging and diseases associated with aging. The alliance can be reached at 2021 K St, N.W., Suite 305, Washington, D. C. 20006; phone 202-293-2856; or fax 202-785-8574.

Eldercare Locator is a service of the National Association of Area Agencies on Aging that provides information about and referrals to respite care and other home and community services offered by State and Area Agencies on Aging. They can be reached at 1112 16th Street, NW, Suite 100, Washington, D. C. 20036, or 800-677-1116.

Alzheimer's Research Centers: The National Institute on Aging funds 28 Alzheimer's Disease Centers (ADCs) at major medical institutions across the country. People at the centers conduct research in all aspects of Alzheimer's disease, with an emphasis on improved care and diagnosis. They also work to train scientists and health care providers who are new to the field. Twenty-seven facilities affiliated with ADCs offer diagnostic and treatment services to patients with Alzheimer's disease and their families. Services and costs vary from facility to facility. For information on individual centers, call or write directly. The centers, and their directors, given in alphabetical order by state, are listed below.

Lindy E. Harrell, M.D., Ph.D.
Department of Neurology
University of Alabama at
    Birmingham
1720 7th Avenue South
Sparks Center 454
Birmingham, **Alabama** 35294-0017
Director: 205-934-3847
Information: 205-934-9775

William J. Jagust, M.D.
Alzheimer's Disease Center
University of California, Davis
Alta Bates Medical Center
2001 Dwight Way
Berkeley, **California** 94704
Director: 510-204-4530

Leon Thal, M.D.
Department of Neuroscience
    (0624)
University of California, San
    Diego School of Medicine
9500 Gilman Drive
La Jolla, **California** 92093-0624
Director: 619-534-4606
Information: 619-622-5800

Jeffrey L. Cummings, M.D.
Department of Neurology and
    Psychiatry
University of California, Los
    Angeles
710 Westwood Plaza
Los Angeles, **California** 90095-1769
Director: 310-206-5238

Caleb E. Finch, Ph.D.
Division of Neurogerontology
Andrus Gerontology Center
University Park, MC-0191
University of Southern California
3715 McClintock Avenue
Los Angeles, **California** 90089-0191
Director: 213-740-1758
Information: 213-740-7777

Suzanne S. Mirra, M.D.
Department of Pathology &
  Laboratory Medicine
Emory University School of
  Medicine
VA Medical Center (151)
1670 Clairmont Road
Decatur, **Georgia** 30033
Director: 404-728-7714

Denis A. Evans, M.D.
Rush Alzheimer's Disease Center
Rush-Presbyterian-St. Lukes
  Medical Center
1645 West Jackson, Suite 675
Chicago, **Illinois** 60612
Director: 312-942-3350
Information: 312-942-4463

Robert E. Becker, M.D.
Center for Alzheimer Disease and
  Related Disorders
Southern Illinois University School
  of Medicine
751 North Rutledge
P.O. Box 19230
Springfield, **Illinois** 62794-1412
Director: 217-785-4468
Information: 217-782-8249 (in IL:
  800-DIAL-SIU)

Bernardino Ghetti, M.D.
Department of Pathology,
  MS-A142
Indiana Alzheimer's Disease
  Center
Indiana University School of
  Medicine
635 Barnhill Drive
Indianapolis, **Indiana** 46202-5120
Director: 317-274-1590
Information: 317-278-2030

William C. Koller, M.D., Ph.D.
Department of Neurology
University of Kansas Medical
  Center
3901 Rainbow Boulevard
Kansas City, **Kansas** 66160-7117
Director: 913-588-6952

William R. Markesbery, M.D.
Sanders-Brown Research Center
  on Aging
University of Kentucky
101 Sanders-Brown Building
800 South Lime
Lexington, **Kentucky** 40536-0230
Director: 606-323-6040

Donald L. Price, M.D.
The Johns Hopkins University
  School of Medicine
558 Ross Research Building
720 Rutland Avenue
Baltimore, **Maryland** 21205
Director: 410-955-5632

John H. Growdon, M.D.
Massachusetts Alzheimer's Disease
Research Center
Massachusetts General Hospital
WAC 830
15 Parkman Street
Boston, **Massachusetts** 02114
Director: 617-726-1728

Sid Gilman, M.D.
Michigan Alzheimer's Disease
Research Center
University of Michigan
1914 Taubman Center
Ann Arbor, **Michigan** 48109-0316
Director: 313-936-9070
Information: 313-764-2190

Ronald Petersen, M.D., Ph.D.
Department of Neurology
Mayo Clinic
200 First Street SW
Rochester, **Minnesota** 55905
Director: 507-284-4006
Information: 507-284-1324

Leonard Berg, M.D.
Alzheimer's Disease Research
Center
Washington University Medical
Center
The Health Key Building
4488 Forest Park Boulevard
St. Louis, **Missouri** 63108-2293
Dir/Information: 314-286-2881

Michael L. Shelanski, M.D., Ph.D.
Alzheimer's Disease Research
Center
Columbia University
630 West 168th Street
New York, **New York** 10032
Director: 212-305-3300
Information: 212-305-8056

Kenneth L. Davis, M.D.
Department of Psychiatry
Mount Sinai School of Medicine
Mount Sinai Medical Center
1 Gustave L. Levy Place,
Box #1230
New York, **New York** 10029-6574
Director: 212-241-6623
Information: 212-241-8329

Steven H. Ferris, Ph.D.
Aging and Dementia Research
Center
New York University Medical
Center, Dept. THN314
550 First Avenue
New York, **New York** 10016
Director: 212-263-5703
Information: 212-263-5700

Paul D. Coleman, Ph.D.
Department of Neurobiology and
Anatomy, Box 603
University of Rochester Medical
Center
601 Elmwood Avenue
Rochester, **New York** 14642
Dir/Information: 716-275-2581

Allen D. Roses, M.D.
Joseph and Kathleen Bryan
  Alzheimer's Disease Research
  Center
Duke University
2200 Main Street, Suite A-230
Durham, **North Carolina** 27705
Dir/Information: 919-286-3228

Peter J. Whitehouse, M.D., Ph.D.
Alzheimer's Disease Center
University Hospitals of Cleveland
11100 Euclid Avenue
Cleveland, **Ohio** 44106
Director: 216-844-7360

Earl A. Zimmerman, M.D.
Department of Neurology (L-226)
Oregon Health Sciences
  University
3181 SW Sam Jackson Park Road
Portland, **Oregon** 97201-3098
Director: 503-494-7321
Information: 503-494-6976

John Q. Trojanowski, M.D., Ph.D.
University of Pennsylvania School
  of Medicine
Room A009, Basement
  Maloney/HUP
36th and Spruce Streets
Philadelphia, **Pennsylvania**
  19104-4283
Director: 215-662-6921
Information: 215-662-6920

Steven DeKosky, M.D.
Alzheimer's Disease Research
  Center
University of Pittsburgh Medical
  Center
Montefiore University Hospital,
  4 West
200 Lothrop Street
Pittsburgh, **Pennsylvania** 15213
Director: 412-624-6889
Information: 412-692-2700

Roger N. Rosenberg, M.D.
Alzheimer's Disease Research
  Center
University of Texas
Southwestern Medical Center at
  Dallas
5323 Harry Hines Boulevard
Dallas, **Texas** 75235-9036
Director: 214-648-3239
Information: 214-648-3198

Stanley H. Appel, M.D.
Alzheimer's Disease Research
  Center
Baylor College of Medicine
6501 Fannin, NB302
Houston, **Texas** 77030-3498
Dir/Information: 713-798-6660

George M. Martin, M.D.
Department of Pathology
University of Washington
Box 357470, HSB K-543
1959 NE Pacific Avenue
Seattle, **Washington** 98195-7470
Director: 206-543-5088
Information: 206-543-6761

Appendix E: The Internet

At publication time for this book, there were several World Wide Web sites that may be useful to people interested in Alzheimer's disease. Washington University (St. Louis, Mo.) has a wonderful e-mail discussion group, called simply "ALZHEIMER," for anyone with an interest in Alzheimer's or related dementing disorders in older adults. The group provides people with different viewpoints an opportunity to share questions, answers, suggestions, and tips. To subscribe to the list, send e-mail to majordomo@wubios.wustl.edu with the message "subscribe alzheimer." You will then receive all messages that are posted to the list. Because the group generates a high volume of postings, you may prefer to receive postings in batches every 2 days or so, in which case you should send the message "subscribe alzheimer-digest" to the same address. You may also send individual questions to ALZHEIMER@wubios.wustl.edu.

Washington University also has good home page and a gopher:

homepage: **http://www.biostat.wustl.edu.alzheimer**
gopher: **gopher://gopher.adrc.wustl.edu**

The Gerontological Society of America has a mailing list called the Informal Interest Group on Alzheimer's Disease Research, which promotes discussions among Alzheimer's disease researchers, educators, and practitioners. If you'd like to be on this mailing list, send e-mail to majordomo @ po.cwru.edu with the command "subscribe gsa-adr (your full e-mail address here)." For further information, contact Jon Stuckey at 216-844-6312.

Another good area to explore is The Massachusetts General Hospital Laboratory of Genetics and Aging Home Page, which can be accessed at the following address:

http://demonmac.mgh.harvard.edu/alzheimers/alzheimer.html

This page has several pointers on it that lead to other valuable sites, some aimed at scientists doing research in the area of Alzheimer's disease (e.g., the "Amyloid Net"), and some designed for interested laypeople, such as the Alzheimer's Association home page, a home page from an Australian Alzheimer's Association, and The Massachusetts General Hospital Neurology Web Forum, where you can ask questions about neurological disorders that will be answered by prominent scientists in each respective area of research. You can access some of the pages connected to this page independently:

The Alzheimer's Association Home Page:
   http://www.alz.org/

The Massachusetts General Hospital Neurology Web Forum:
   http://demonmac.mgh.harvard.edu/neurowebforum/
   neurowebforum.html

The Alzheimer's Web Home Page (from Australia):
   http://werple.mira.net.au/%7Edhs/ad.html

In addition, you may want to try some of the following:

The Alzheimer's Bookshelf:
   http://www.nbn.com/people/elder/
   alzheimer.html

The Indiana Alzheimer Disease Center National Cell Repository:
   http://medgen.iupui.edu/-medgen/research/alzheimer/

ADEAR's web page:
   http://www.alzheimers.org/adear

Notes

1. G. McKhann, D. Drachman, M. Folstein, et al., "Clinical Diagnosis of Alzheimer's Disease: Report of the NINCDS-ADRDA Work Group," *Neurology* 34 (1984): 939–44.

2. Marcia Barinaga, "New Alzheimer's Gene Found," *Science* 268 (1995): 1845–46; and Marcia Barinaga, "Missing Alzheimer's Gene Found," *Science* 269 (1995): 91–92. These brief news pieces describe the discovery of the Alzheimer-associated genes S182 and STM2 and clarify how their discovery fits into existing knowledge about genetic causes of Alzheimer's disease.

3. G. W. Small, J. C. Mazziota, M. T. Collins, et al., "Apolipoprotein E Type 4 Allele and Cerebral Glucose Metabolism in Relatives at Risk for Familial Alzheimer's Disease," *Journal of the American Medical Association* 273 (1995): 942–47.

4. Readers who want to learn more details of the relationship between the APO E genes and Alzheimer's disease may want to look up M. I. Kamboh, "Apolipoprotein E Polymorphism and Susceptibility to Alzheimer's Disease," *Human Biology* 67 (1995): 195–215. Considering the technical nature of its subject matter, this review article is quite accessible and will serve to provide more in-depth analysis of what is now known on this subject.

5. Scientists of the American College of Medical Genetics/American Society of Human Genetics Working Group on APO E and Alzheimer's Disease came to a consensus in 1995 that, though the presence of the APO E4 gene is strongly associated with Alzheimer's disease, at the present time APO E genetic testing is not recommended for use in routine clinical diagnosis. *Journal of the American Medical Association* 274 (1995): 1627–29.

6. Where the genotyping for apolipoprotein E *is* available, it is quite expensive. For example, at Specialty Laboratories, Inc., in Santa Monica, California, the cost of analysis is $160 *in addition* to the costs of blood collection and sample preparation.

7. L. F. M. Scinto, K. R. Daffner, D. Dressler, B. I. Ransil, D. Rentz, S. Weintraub, M. Mesulam, H. Potter, "A Potential Noninvasive

Neurobiological Test for Alzheimer's Disease," *Science* 266 (1994): 1051–54.

8. R. Etcheberrigaray, E. Ito, K. Oka, B. Tofel-Grehl, G. E. Gibson, D. L. Alkon, "Potassium Channel Dysfunction in Fibroblasts Identifies Patients with Alzheimer Disease," *Proceedings of the National Academy of Sciences* 90 (1993): 8209–13.

9. N. Pomara, M. Stanley, P. A. LeWitt, et al., "Increased CSF HVA Response to Arecoline Challenge in Alzheimer's Disease," *Journal of Neural Transmission, General Section* 90 (1992): 53–65.

Index

Attorney, power of. *See* Power of attorney

Autopsy: diagnosis, 7, 11; importance, 40, 47; limitations, 46

Aventyl, 81, 118

Axon, 22, 40, 42; illus., 23; length, 22; sending message, 24

Azapirone, 119

B12, vitamin, 86

Bank accounts, 71; transfer of authority, 73

Bathing, 61

Bathroom: restlessness and, 62; sexually explicit behaviors and, 65; simplifying use of, 62; wandering and, 63–64

Behavior changes: as measure of improvement in clinical trials, 93; in multi-infarct dementia, 8; in Pick's disease, 9; universality of, in Alzheimer's disease, 79

Behavior problems, 6, 62–65; handling, 62–65, 79

Behavioral symptoms, assessing, 16

Benjamin B. Green-Field National Alzheimer's Library and Resource Center, 125

Benzodiazepines, 119

Besipirdine, 101

Beta amyloid, 47; accumulation of, 35, 103; binding to apolipoprotein E, 43; in transgenic mice, 89; involvement in neural damage, 42, 103,

105; production of, 34, 42, 89; promotion of growth by apolipoprotein E4, 106; S182 and, 35; spurring production of apolipoprotein E, 43. *See also* Amyloid

Bethanechol, 99

Blessed Dementia Rating Scale, 16

Blood, clots, 18; tests, 15; vessel damage, 18

Blood pressure: high, 93; as side effect, 118; history of, 14; medications for, 82; risk for multi-infarct dementia, 8; low, 84

Blood-brain barrier, 103–04; gangliosides and, 108; nerve growth factor and, 107

Brain, 22–25; abnormalities in Alzheimer's disease, 40; disorders, 117; injury of, as dementia cause, 10; neurons in, 22; onset of changes in, 49, 95, 114; tumors, 15, 18. *See also* Brain scans

Brain scans, 17–20, 26; in diagnosis, 10, 97; misinterpretation of, 10. *See also* Computed tomography; Magnetic resonance imaging; Positron emission tomography; Single-photon emission computed tomography

Bupropion, 81, 118

Buspar, 82, 119

Buspirone, 82, 119